CH00670005

Mental Health and Digestion

Breaking Free From Emotional Struggles through Gut Health

D. R. Darcy

© Copyright 2023 - All rights reserved.

The content contained within this book may not be reproduced, duplicated or transmitted without direct written permission from the author or the publisher.

Under no circumstances will any blame or legal responsibility be held against the publisher, or author, for any damages, reparation, or monetary loss due to the information contained within this book, either directly or indirectly.

Legal Notice:

This book is copyright protected. It is only for personal use. You cannot amend, distribute, sell, use, quote or paraphrase any part, or the content within this book, without the consent of the author or publisher.

Disclaimer Notice:

Please note the information contained within this document is for educational and entertainment purposes only. All effort has been executed to present accurate, up to date, reliable, complete information. No warranties of any kind are declared or implied. Readers acknowledge that the author is not engaged in the rendering of legal, financial, medical or professional advice. The content within this book has been derived from various sources. Please consult a licensed professional before attempting any techniques outlined in this book.

By reading this document, the reader agrees that under no circumstances is the author responsible for any losses, direct or indirect, that are incurred as a result of the use of the information contained within this document, including, but not limited to, errors, omissions, or inaccuracies.

Table of Contents

Introduction:

Unleashing the Power Within:

Cultivating Emotional Wellness

Through Gut Health

I'm not the kind of guy who likes to make his opinion known in every room he walks into. In fact, I prefer one-on-one conversations where I can gather information and then give my opinion accordingly. So, it was slightly out of character when I turned to the two ladies behind me in line at the grocery store. Despite the internal war that raged moments earlier between my eagerness to help and my restrictiveness to give an opinion when it wasn't asked, I finally mustered up the courage to talk to them. "Excuse me, I couldn't help but overhear your conversation," I said as politely as possible, totally aware of the fact that that might sound slightly creepy. "Are either of you struggling with severe anxiety?" One of the ladies nodded, then quickly added that they weren't interested in buying any supplements from me that might help them. I couldn't help but laugh as I quickly explained that I wasn't in the business of selling some sort of magical supplement. Instead, I asked another question, risking the possibility of offending them. "If you don't mind me asking, how's your digestion?" The lady looked at me as if I just asked her whether she had ever been to Mars. "Well, not that it's any of your business," she said defensively, but then her expression softened. "But yes, I struggle severely with my digestion."

I wasn't surprised by her shock, and I also wasn't surprised by her answers. We spent the next five minutes holding up the line and discussing the connection between her gut and her mental health. At first, she was skeptical, but the more I shared with her about the journey I've been on and the research I've been doing, the more she relaxed and asked questions. By the end of the conversation, she turned to her friend and told her that she would have to add some different foods to her cart, and as she walked away, she smiled at me, thanked me, and said, "You should write a book about this. I know I would benefit from it, and so would many other people I know." I thanked her, paid for my groceries, and started making my way home. Yet, I couldn't shake the idea. *"Perhaps I should write a book?"* I wondered. Well, after months of additional research, here I am, writing a book for that kind lady in the supermarket, as well as for you, dear reader.

I've traveled the world, and there are two things that I always encounter, no matter where I go: emotional distress and digestive issues. So, it came as no surprise when I learned that the two are actually very closely connected to one another, and it all starts with something that we call *the gut-brain axis*. The gut-brain axis is a complex network of communication between the brain and the gastrointestinal tract. It connects the systems, making it a two-way communication method between the gut and the brain. There are many components to the gut-brain axis which we'll discuss over the course of this book, but for now, all you need to come to terms with is the fact that these two concepts are very closely connected. Your mental health, mood, and thinking have a massive impact on your digestive system and vice versa. As bizarre as it might sound, stick with me, and I promise that by the end of this book, it will all make sense.

Now, my goal for you on this journey isn't just to learn theory. As great as knowledge and theory are, they don't really change your life much. No, if we want theory to be meaningful, it needs to move into action. That's why this book will be filled with a combination of theory and practice. Not only will we learn how things work, but we'll also learn what to do about these things and how to make lasting changes that will benefit us from the inside out. The gut-brain axis includes digestive function, mood regulation, immunity, and pain management. It controls so many aspects of your body that contribute to the way you live your life. That's why we need to take action and not only fix our relationship with our minds and our bodies as two separate entities but transform the way we view these two aspects of our lives altogether. However, before we jump into anything else, there are a few foundational aspects that we need to cover in the Introduction.

Your brain and your gut are connected both physically and biochemically, which means that poor gut health can lead to mental health disorders such as depression and anxiety. Luckily, the opposite is also true. When you have a healthy gut, you will experience reduced stress, mood regulation, enhanced cognitive function, and better resilience to emotional challenges. However, we shouldn't forget that the communication line goes both ways. The state of your mental health also influences the state of your gut. So, if you have poor mental health, you are more likely to struggle with digestive issues, and when you have good mental health, your digestive tract should respond accordingly. It's a little bit like the chicken and the egg conundrum. We don't really know which came first, but we know that they are now in a continuous cycle. Whether you first encounter issues with your gut due to unhealthy eating habits or an unhealthy relationship with food, or whether you first experienced anxiety or stress, the two will ultimately influence one another and cause the other to respond. Luckily, since we now have the knowledge of this cycle, we get to stop it and flip it so that they can influence one another positively instead of negatively. The question is: how? How can we stop the cycle and put it in reverse to work in our favor instead of against us? Well, that's what I'm here for, and that's where the practical side of this book will kick in!

Before we take a single step further, I first want to put you at ease by saying that this is a judgment-free zone. My gut health has been a mess before, and so has my mental health. I have no intention of making you feel guilty for experiencing these issues. In fact, I want you to feel like I'm your biggest supporter and that I'm in your corner, rooting for you! So, try to show yourself that same courtesy. As we journey through these pages, you might read something and realize, "Man, I haven't been taking very good care of my mental health," but instead of feeling guilty about it, I want you to feel empowered. Use that realization as fuel to incorporate change instead of seeing it as something you need to feel bad about. Do we have a deal? Instead of focusing on the things you might have neglected in the past, see this as an opportunity to improve your tomorrow. Beating yourself up will not only make you feel miserable, but it will also be counterproductive since that will then affect both your mental and gut health as a result.

So, what exactly will we cover on this journey? Well, let's have a closer look at what we'll explore in every chapter.

- In Chapter 1, we'll look at the gut microbiome, and start to see how this microbiome affects our emotional well-being. We'll also use the opportunity to identify possible areas that we can improve on to boost the health of our gut microbiome. Practically, we'll look at how we can use our gut to improve our mental well-being.

- Chapter 2 is all about gut memory. I know it might sound weird to think that your gut has a memory, but this is where I expect you'll have many light bulb moments. We'll look at understanding PTSD and how it can affect your gut, as well as strategies to combat PTSD.

- When talking about the gut and the mind, we also need to address hormones and the role they play in both of these areas. In Chapter 3, we'll look at hormones and how an imbalance in hormones can cause serious harm to both your gut and your emotional well-being. We'll look at lifestyle strategies to combat hormonal imbalance as well as other strategies to improve hormone well-being.

- In Chapter 4, we'll look at how we can ease our anxiety since it has such a significant influence on our health. We'll look at a couple of techniques to deal with anxiety and practices that will help us gain a new perspective on anxiety and nutrition.

- Vitamins can turn some of the darkest times into lighter ones, so in Chapter 5, we'll look at the role of vitamins on mental health and which vitamins we should be sure to include in order to maintain a healthy mindset.

- Chapter 6 is all about embracing inner peace and managing stress levels by taking good care of the gut. We'll explore various techniques that can be useful to achieve inner peace, such as art and journaling. We'll also look at how we can use stress to our advantage and make the most of a bad situation.

- In Chapter 7, I'll encourage you to take a good, long nap! We'll talk about the importance of rest and how sleep can contribute to healthy emotional well-being as well as a healthy gut. We'll discuss a couple of important sleep hygiene techniques that you can implement immediately.

- Emotional eating plays a huge role in both gut health and mental health, which is why Chapter 8 is dedicated to addressing emotional eating and finding healthy solutions for it. We'll dive a little deeper into understanding emotional eating as well as identifying triggers that might prompt emotional eating.

- Chapter 9 will address movement and how it can contribute to a healthier gut and increased emotional well-being. We'll explore different types of exercises that are beneficial for gut and emotional health, as well as how to find joy in movement (yes, it can be fun)!

- In our final chapter, we'll explore the longevity and sustainability of these practical changes. Unlike a three-week diet that's not sustainable at all, these changes should contribute to the well-being of all ages and increase gut health regardless of how old you are.

As you can see, this journey is packed with both theory and practice, which is why I am confident that it will be incredibly beneficial to you. Remember, there's no judgment here, so it doesn't matter what the state of your mental or gut health is right now; you're in the right place. I can't wait to continue on this journey with you—and just know that I will be here with you every single step of the way.

Chapter 1:

The Gut Microbiome:

Illuminating the Path to

Emotional Well-Being

Have you ever heard someone refer to your gut as your second brain? While that might sound strange, it's actually not as inaccurate as we might think. The gut microbiome is a collection of trillions of microorganisms that live in your gut. These microorganisms are also known as bacteria, fungi, protozoa, and even viruses. They play an essential role in your overall well-being—and not just your digestive system but also your emotional well-being. Don't worry, though, your gut was made for all these microorganisms, and they're not all harmful. In fact, many of them are necessary for daily functions. The gut microbiome is unique in every person, and there are many factors that influence your gut microbiome. That's why it can lead to various illnesses and diseases for different people. An unhealthy gut microbiome can lead to obesity, inflammation, and allergies. Your gut microbiome is also a source of protection since it is responsible for more than half of your immune system.

While all of this is great to know, there's another interesting fact about the gut microbiome that often gets overlooked, which I believe is the most crucial aspect of all: The gut microbiome can influence your mood, behavior, and thoughts. Yes, you read that right! Your gut can quite literally influence your mental health, which means that your gut can be the key to emotional well-being. Since your gut can influence your mental health negatively, it should also be able to influence it positively. However, that requires some work and being intentional with our gut health. In this chapter, we'll look at the complicated relationship between gut and emotional well-being. In order to successfully find strategies to combat mental health-related problems through a healthy gut, we first need to understand how these concepts are connected. Once we have a better understanding of the complicated relationship, we'll look at how to unleash the power from within and use our gut health to promote emotional well-being. We'll also look at strategies and remedies that we can incorporate to ensure that we have a healthy gut and a healthy mind.

I want to encourage you to approach this chapter with an open mind and make notes of the questions that you might have. Some of the topics we'll only touch on now and dive in deeper later, so be sure to note when something piques your interest or if you read something that really stands out for you. The more actively you participate as we journey through these pages, the more beneficial it will be for you. With that being said, let's have a look at the complicated relationship of your gut and your mind.

The Complicated Relationship

Your gut microbiome affects your emotional well-being through the production of neurotransmitters. Neurotransmitters are chemicals that act as messengers between your nerve cells. Neurotransmitters are in charge of regulating your mood, managing behavior, and many other functions. Many neurotransmitters are produced by the gut, including hormones such as serotonin, dopamine, and gamma-aminobutyric (GABA). You might recognize some of these names since serotonin and dopamine are often referred to as happy hormones. This is how we can already start to see how a healthy gut can influence your mental health.

There are many different types of microbiomes that live in the gut, and they have various functions. Let's have a look at some of the most common microbiomes and how they contribute to our overall well-being and health (Valdes et al., 2018).

- **Bifidobacterium:** These bacteria are known for their ability to produce short-chain fatty acids. These fatty acids contribute to your health by reducing inflammation and improving your gut barrier.

- **Lactobacillus:** These bacteria have the ability to break down lactose and other complex carbohydrates.

- **Bacteroides:** This is the type of bacteria that are the most abundant in most people's gut, and their primary purpose is to digest fiber.

- **Enterococcus:** These bacteria protect your gut from harmful bacteria and they produce vitamins.

- **Escherichia coli:** These bacteria help your body to digest food and process vitamins that your body requires to function.

When your gut microbiome is balanced and healthy, it will actively work to reduce inflammation in your body. High levels of inflammation are known to contribute to chronic diseases such as anxiety and depression. Therefore, if your gut is healthy, your brain has a better shot at also being healthy. When your gut is less diverse than it should be, meaning that it has fewer good bacteria present, you are more likely to experience anxiety and depression. It will be much harder for you to regulate your emotional well-being and mood due to the lack of gut bacteria. When your gut isn't operating at the level it should, adding probiotic supplements can help to reduce your anxiety symptoms, as well as improve your overall mood.

To recap what we've learned, we now know that your gut and brain are connected to one another, and if one is suffering, so will the other. However, if one is thriving, the other will respond accordingly. That's why we can use our gut to improve our mindset and mental health, working from the inside out.

Unleashing the Power Within

In order to make your gut work for you in a positive way and contribute to mental well-being, you need first to be aware of how to take proper care of your gut. When you take good care of your gut, you instinctively take a step toward better overall health since your gut contributes to various areas of your mind and body. The most obvious way that we can take care of our gut is by looking at our diet and determining whether our diet is contributing to our health or placing stress on our gut. When looking at your diet, there are five specifics that you need to consider.

Balanced Diet

If you want to have a healthy gut, the first question you need to ask yourself is whether you are eating and maintaining a balanced diet. A balanced diet doesn't mean eating only salads and locking away the cookies forever. In fact, if you only eat lettuce and celery, your diet won't be very balanced either. A balanced diet is when you provide your body with all the essential nutrients in order to function correctly. This includes eating a variety of protein, fat, fiber, vitamins, minerals, and carbohydrates. Although some diets make it seem as if carbohydrates and fat are villains, they are actually essential for your well-being. A balanced diet also includes eating the correct portion sizes. Since we're all different and our guts work in unique ways, my portion size might be different than yours; that is why it's essential that you listen to your body when it comes to fullness and hunger. If you want to have a balanced diet, you should learn to eat until you are full and then stop. Eating too little might lead to binge eating later, and overeating will place a lot of pressure on your gut. Here are a few ways that you can incorporate a balanced diet:

- Eat loads of fruits and vegetables.

- Include lean protein in your diet.

- Stay hydrated by drinking eight glasses of water a day.

Limiting Processed Food

Another way that you can take care of your gut health is by limiting processed food. Even though a majority of food in most supermarkets is highly processed, you should try to limit how often you consume processed foods such as meats and canned goods. I suggest reading the labels on the food items to educate yourself on what you're actually putting into your body. Instead of consuming loads of processed foods, try to make use of fresh ingredients that you can get at local markets. Or better yet, if you have the facilities to do so, you can start your own garden at home. While removing all processed foods is nearly impossible, the goal is simply to prioritize fresh produce and not eliminate processed foods completely. You can limit processed foods by

- cooking at home instead of eating takeout meals.

- reading the labels carefully before purchasing ingredients.

- stocking your pantry with healthy snacks instead of processed goods.

Fiber-Rich Foods

It's essential not only to focus on removing certain things from your diet but also to add certain foods in order to ensure a healthy gut. One thing that you should add to your meals is foods that are high in fiber. When meals are high in fiber, you will feel more satisfied with the meal since it contributes to feeling full. Fiber also helps regulate bowel movements, and it lowers the risk of chronic diseases such as heart disease, stroke, and type 2 diabetes. There are many ways that you can add more fiber to your diet, such as

- eating a hearty breakfast that is high in fiber, such as oatmeal or whole-wheat toast.

- adding beans and lentils to your plate since they are great sources of fiber and protein.

- including vegetables in all your meals since they are a great source of fiber.

Fermented Foods

Fermented foods are often overlooked when the topic of gut health is approached. However, fermented foods can help your gut to manage bacteria. Fermented foods are foods that have been preserved through fermentation, which includes the use of bacteria or yeast to break down sugars and starches. Fermented foods have been part of the human diet for centuries, and they are still highly beneficial for all. Fermented foods include the following:

- yogurt

- kefir

- sauerkraut

- kimchi

- tempeh

- miso

- kombucha

Fermented foods are great for your gut health because they contain probiotics. Probiotics improve your digestion, boost your immune system, and protect against chronic diseases. Probiotics help the gut to function, and they restore the balance of the bacteria within your gut. Probiotics also contribute to a healthy immune system, which allows your gut to function effectively. Adding fermented foods to your diet can be quite tricky, especially if you're not used to the taste. However, they're essential for a healthy gut. Here are a couple of ways that you can start adding fermented foods to your diet:

- Start with small amounts and work your way up from there.

- Choose a variety of foods so that you can get the most benefits from them.

- Look for foods that are made with live cultures.

- Be sure to store the fermented foods properly in order to remain fresh.

- Listen to your body so that if you experience a highly upset gut after consuming fermented foods, you can reduce your intake.

Prebiotics

While fermented foods make use of probiotics, prebiotics are equally as important. Prebiotics are nondigestible food ingredients that are beneficial for your gut health. They are a type of fiber that activates your gut and are beneficial for gut health. Prebiotics improve your gut health by feeding the probiotics in your gut. When probiotics consume prebiotics, they produce even more fatty acids that have a beneficial effect on your body. Prebiotics also promote the growth of beneficial bacteria, which improves not only your digestion but your overall health. Prebiotics also inhibit the growth of harmful bacteria and protect the body against infections. There are many types of prebiotics, and many foods naturally contain prebiotics. These foods include

- onions

- garlic

- leeks

- asparagus

- chickpeas

- beans

- whole grains

Similarly to probiotics, if you are new to consuming prebiotics, start off nice and slow and add it to your diet one ingredient at a time. You might experience some digestive upset the first couple of times that you consume prebiotics, but it should settle within the first couple of days.

Now that we have a better idea of how to improve our gut from the inside out in order to influence our mindset positively, there are also other approaches to boosting your gut health that go beyond just your meals. These ingredients are often viewed as a more holistic approach to gut health since they don't only affect your gut but also other health-related issues. In the next section, we'll take a look at a couple of holistic approaches to positively take care of your gut health without introducing you to foreign concepts. So, if you feel intimidated by the word *holistic*, don't worry! I promise I won't introduce you to anything that might make you feel uncomfortable.

The Holistic Approach

Holistic remedies refer to additional approaches to healing your gut that don't include medication or doctor appointments. While talking to your doctor or local pharmacist isn't a bad idea, some people prefer a more natural approach when it comes to taking care of their gut. These holistic remedies are all-natural ingredients that you can consume that will contribute to your gut health. While there are various holistic ingredients that you can choose from, these five, in particular, are my favorites.

Chamomile

Chamomile is a flowering plant that has been used for centuries in treating different medical conditions. This plant contains antioxidants which makes it a great natural course of treatment for many. Chamomile also contains anti-inflammatory, antibacterial, and antispasmodic properties, which boost your overall health and well-being. For this reason, chamomile is an excellent holistic remedy for healing your gut. Chamomile can help your gut heal in the following ways:

- **Reducing inflammation:** Since chamomile contains anti-inflammatory properties, it reduces the levels of inflammation in your gut which is often the cause of pain. Chamomile is a great option if you struggle with irritable bowel syndrome.

- **Promoting gut healing:** Chamomile promotes healing within your gut lining, which is essential when restoring your gut. When your gut lining has been damaged, you might experience diseases such as leaky gut and other gut-related issues.

- **Reducing gut bacteria:** When you consume chamomile, it reduces the risk of harmful bacteria in your gut. When you have less harmful bacteria, your gut will start to improve its health.

- **Improving digestion:** Chamomile is known to also help aid in digestion by relaxing the muscles in your gut. When your gut muscles are tense, you might start to experience constipation and other discomfort in the gut area. By releasing the tension of those muscles, you actively work against the tension that your gut might experience.

- **Reducing stress:** Chamomile works as a great stress reliever, and since stress impacts your gut, chamomile also prevents your gut from taking damage when you relax and destress.

The most common and popular way of consuming chamomile is by drinking chamomile tea, but there are also other ways that you can add chamomile to your diet. You can also add chamomile as an ingredient to your food, such as in soups and stews. Chamomile is also available in tablets that you can purchase at most health stores. If you're not interested in consuming chamomile, you can also try to apply it topically to reduce inflammation and irritation. You can purchase chamomile cream at most health food stores or at pharmacies.

Peppermint

Another popular holistic remedy is peppermint. Peppermint is a herb that has been used for centuries to treat digestive problems. Peppermint is often prescribed to fight indigestion, nausea, and diarrhea. Another popular use for peppermint is in managing irritable bowel syndrome symptoms. The reason why peppermint is so effective is due to the active ingredient menthol. Menthol has antispasmodic and anti-inflammatory properties, which provide the muscles in your gut with relaxation properties. Peppermint also increases the production of mucus in the gut, which protects the lining of the gut better.

According to a study conducted in 2020, peppermint oil can significantly reduce the symptoms of IBS. The same study found that peppermint oil can be used to reduce abdominal pain, bloating, and flatulence (Ried et al., 2020). Peppermint doesn't only come in oil form, though—it can be used in a variety of ways, including tablets, teas, and capsules. You can use peppermint in the following ways:

- **Peppermint tea:** Peppermint tea is a delicious and easy way to reap the benefits of the herb. It's also inexpensive and easily accessible.

- **Peppermint capsules:** If you're not interested in drinking tea, you can opt for peppermint capsules which are very convenient. Peppermint tablets can be found at most health stores.

- **Peppermint essential oil:** If you don't want to consume tea, you can also add peppermint oil to some hot water or to your food. You can also apply peppermint oil topically if you don't want to consume it.

Peppermint is safe to use, and it is a very effective way of taking good care of your gut. However, peppermint can cause heartburn or acid reflux for some people, so if you experience those symptoms, try one of the other remedies instead or speak to your local healthcare provider.

Ginger

Another herb that has been used for centuries is ginger. Ginger is known for its anti-inflammatory properties, but it can also aid in digestion and provide antioxidants. Ginger can potentially help your gut in various ways that are beneficial to your gut as well as your mind. Ginger contains all the same benefits as chamomile, in other words, it

- reduces inflammation.

- protects your gut lining.

- improves digestion.

- reduces nausea and vomiting.

Ginger can be slightly trickier to add to your daily meals since it has a stronger taste and flavor than chamomile and peppermint. However, certain people truly love the taste of ginger, which makes this the ideal holistic remedy. If you want to start adding ginger to your meals, be sure to start with a small amount of ginger and increase the amount over a period of time, allowing your body to get used to it. If you experience any side effects such as diarrhea or heartburn, stop consuming the ginger and speak to your healthcare provider about it. It's essential that you store ginger in a cool dry place so that it can last longer and keep its medicinal value. Ginger is considered a fairly safe herb to consume, so if you have gut issues, this is a great herb to try first.

Lavender

Next, we're looking at lavender. While most people know lavender as a scent or flavoring, this small flower really packs a punch! Lavender has a calming effect on your body and mind, and it improves the growth of your gut health. Lavender contains similar properties to other herbs, such as anti-inflammatory compounds and antioxidants. The great thing about lavender is that it is a stress reducer, so your gut should be able to relax more when you're making use of lavender. There are many different ways that we can benefit from lavender, all pretty similar to chamomile and peppermint. When you decide what you want to use, you can drink lavender tea, take lavender oil, or use lavender oil in a diffuser. Lavender is generally a safe herb, but I recommend you speak to your healthcare provider before making any big changes to your diet. One of my favorite drinks is lavender tea, and I drink a cup before bed every night since it helps me to relax and sleep well.

Lemon

Lemons are a great source of fiber, which can help improve gut health. Fiber can also slow down the digestion of sugars and starches, which prevents spikes in your blood sugar levels while allowing for more regular energy boosts. Lemons also contain pectin, which is a type of fiber that promotes the growth of bacteria in the gut. When you consume pectin, the healthy bacteria in your gut will grow and restore the balance within the gut lining. Lemon is also known to help prevent gut digestion issues, such as diarrhea, constipation, and irritable bowel syndrome. Another wonderful characteristic of lemon is that it contains loads of vitamin C, which is an antioxidant that can protect your gut lining from damage. Vitamin C is absolutely essential in the production of collagen, which is a protein that keeps the gut healthy.

While it might be tricky to eat a lemon due to its sour nature, there are other ways that you can add lemon to your diet, such as

- adding lemon to your water by squeezing half a lemon into your glass.

- adding lemon to your food by using the juices in your salad, vegetables, and fish.

- making lemon tea by adding a couple of slices of lemon to hot water and allowing it to brew for a couple of minutes.

- making lemon balm by stewing lemon leaves in hot water and then consuming it like tea.

Lemons are a great option to improve your gut health in a natural way, and lemons are easily accessible and affordable to most. These holistic remedies can greatly contribute to your gut health, which indirectly also contributes to your mental health. However, when it comes to taking good care of your gut, it goes beyond just adding additional things to your diet or limiting other types of foods. That's because if you want a healthy gut, you need to embrace a lifestyle that contributes to and cultivates a healthy gut. Let's have a look at what it means to embrace a healthy gut lifestyle.

Embracing a Gut-Healthy Lifestyle

Your gut is essential for your overall health and well-being, so it's almost unfair to expect a couple of added ingredients to do the trick and make your gut run smoothly again. That's why you need to embrace a lifestyle that contributes to a healthy gut and not just rely on what you eat or don't eat. Remember, your gut is connected to your mind and emotions, so if you want to take proper care of your gut, you also need to take care of the other areas. As we look at a couple of ways that we can embrace a gut-healthy lifestyle, keep in mind that we'll be touching on these topics in much greater detail in future chapters. However, for now, see these points as a bit of an introduction or sneak peek of what's to come. There are four vital elements to embracing a gut-healthy lifestyle which are self-care, stress management, deep breathing exercises, and proper sleep hygiene. Let's have a closer look at each of these areas.

Self-Care

Self-care is one of those topics that is often misunderstood. I am also guilty of this! For a very long time, I believed that self-care was just another word for acting selfishly or being self-absorbed. In truth, self-care is actually quite the opposite of that. Put plainly, and I hope you'd agree: We simply should never feel guilty about taking care of ourselves. It's funny to think about it, really. Self-care is the act of taking care of your personal needs in order for you to be your best self. If you neglect your own needs, you can't possibly give others the best of what you have. There's this saying that I absolutely love that goes, "You can't pour from an empty cup." When you don't take care of yourself and fill your own cup, you won't be able to give others what they deserve. If you want others to experience who you truly are and gift them your time and love, you need to be the best version of yourself in order to do so, which is only possible by taking time to care for yourself. There are numerous ways that you can practice self-care, and depending on your needs, it might look different from person to person. We'll explore how we can use self-care to heal from post-traumatic stress disorder in Chapter 2, and we'll look at some other practical emotional self-care examples in Chapter 8, but for now, I want to look at all the different types of self-care that you can find and the areas that you can start prioritizing in your life. These include

- physical self-care, which includes movement, a healthy diet, and getting enough sleep.

- mental self-care, which includes relaxing, spending time in nature, and journaling.

- emotional self-care, which includes expressing emotions, taking time for yourself, and saying no to things you don't have time for.

- spiritual self-care, which includes connecting to a faith, practicing gratitude, and helping others.

- social self-care, which includes spending time with loved ones, joining a club, and volunteering your time.

- professional self-care, which includes setting boundaries, taking breaks, and learning new skills.

- financial self-care, which includes budgeting, saving, and investing.

When you practice self-care regularly, your physical and emotional well-being will benefit from it, and your gut will be better off as well. Self-care contributes to gut health by focusing and prioritizing activities that will actively contribute toward your well-being.

Stress Reduction Techniques

Embracing a lifestyle that promotes good gut health requires you to practice stress reduction techniques. Our lives are filled with stressors that influence our gut health negatively, and even though we can't do much to control the stress in the world that we have to deal with, we can control whether we do something to get rid of the stress or not. Even though stress and anxiety have become very normalized, you don't have to allow stress to take over your whole world. Instead, you dedicate time toward stress reduction techniques such as exercise, spending time in nature, and being mindful. We'll look at stress reduction techniques in further chapters as well, so we won't get into specifics right now. However, right now it's vital for you to decide that you are willing to dedicate time in your schedule to get rid of the stress in your life. If you want a healthy gut, you should prioritize dealing with the emotional side effects of chronic stress and take precautionary steps to avoid falling into burnout and other emotional stressors.

Deep Breathing

One of the stress reduction strategies that can improve your gut health immediately is learning how to breathe deeply. Deep breathing is a simple, yet effective way that you can use to reduce stress by sending the appropriate signals to your body and mind. The signals that get transported when you practice deep breathing communicate to your mind and body that you are safe and that it's okay to relax. When you're constantly stressed, your gut muscles will tense up, and this will slow down your metabolism which can cause additional issues. Deep breathing is a simple act, and taking a couple of minutes a day to focus on your breathing can contribute greatly to your overall health and well-being.

As we reach the end of this chapter, I want to encourage you to process everything you've read so far. Then, think about what practice or technique you can start implementing today that will promote your gut health and mental health. It doesn't have to be something big or time-consuming—keep it simple and attainable. This is your first practical step on this glorious journey, and only you can implement these changes into your life. In the next chapter, we'll look at how your gut has a memory and how emotional wounds and PTSD can contribute to gut-related issues.

Chapter 2:

Gut Memory and PTSD:

Healing the Emotional Wounds

A good friend of mine spent 10 years in the military. She saw and experienced some unthinkable things, including friends getting shot right next to her. After her tenth year in the military, she went home and started having flashbacks and nightmares of the times spent in the military. She often woke up in the middle of the night, drenched in sweat, with her heart racing a thousand miles a minute. Slowly, she started isolating herself and avoiding people in order to avoid talking about her issues and her time in the military. After a couple of months of barely any sleep, she was diagnosed with post-traumatic stress disorder (PTSD). This is a very common occurrence for people who have experienced trauma, as she did in the military. Along with the nightmares, she also experienced gut issues for the first time in her life.

Eventually, my friend spoke to her therapist who explained to her that her gut was struggling because of gut memory. Gut memory happens when you have trapped emotions in your brain and body that live in your subconscious mind. However, even when the trauma is in your subconscious, your body becomes aware of it, especially your gut. My friend realized that she had to take care of her gut and in order to do so, she would have to face her PTSD and release some of the hidden emotions.

While my friend was able to recognize she had PTSD, many of us don't acknowledge that we're suffering from it. When you serve in the military or experience other types of obvious trauma, PTSD is usually a topic that a healthcare provider will bring up with you. However, for many of us, we carry small traumas in our gut that appear so insignificant that we don't address them, but they can influence our entire well-being, especially our gut. In this chapter, we'll look at what post-traumatic stress disorder is and how we can manage it better with a psychological approach. We'll also look at some strategies for dealing with PTSD and look at a holistic approach to recovering from trauma in your life. Most of us experience trauma somewhere in our lives. While some trauma is more obvious (like watching someone die), other trauma is less obvious, like harboring a fear of rejection because your mom forgot to pick you up from school when you were 10. So, don't assume that PTSD-related content won't be applicable to you. You might just be surprised at how much you'll be able to learn about yourself and your hidden emotions.

What Is Post-Traumatic Stress Disorder?

Post-traumatic stress disorder is a mental health condition that people develop after experiencing or witnessing a life-threatening event. This includes natural disasters, combat, a car accident, or sexual assault (NCCIH, 2020). In the wake of a traumatic event, upsetting memories are common, as are generally feeling on edge, and, of course, having issues with sleep. That being said, feelings like these typically disappear after a couple of weeks. When these feelings don't go away, it might be due to PTSD. Every person experiences PTSD in their own way since everyone's trauma is different from one another. However, there are a couple of common PTSD symptoms that remain constant, which include

- reliving the event through flashbacks and nightmares.

- avoiding anything that might remind you of the event.

- experiencing negative changes in mood.

- feeling detached from reality.

- noticing changes in physical reaction such as being startled easily or being annoyed with others.

PTSD can be hazardous both to you and those around you, but it's essential that you remember you're not alone and that together we can find a solution to ease the PTSD symptoms. Trauma can have a big impact on the gut-brain axis since it triggers a fight-or-flight response in your body and mind. Trauma disrupts the bacteria in your gut and can cause your gut to become inflamed. Not all trauma affects your brain and gut the same way, and there are even different kinds of PTSD.

- **Uncomplicated PTSD:** This is the most common type of PTSD, and it is caused by one single traumatic event, such as a natural disaster or assault.

- **Complex PTSD:** Complex PTSD is caused by prolonged or repeated exposure to trauma, like being abused consistently as a child or in military combat.

- **Delayed-onset PTSD:** Delayed-onset PTSD is trauma that develops years after the traumatic event. This is mainly due to hidden emotions that only surface years after in order to keep you safe.

- **Vicarious trauma PTSD:** Vicarious trauma happens when you witness or hear about a traumatic event that happened to someone else that greatly affects you.

- **Secondary PTSD:** Secondary PTSD can come from taking care of someone else who has PTSD. By taking care of the other person, you experience their trauma as if it were your own since you can see the aftermath of the trauma.

Over the years, there have been various treatment plans to help people who are suffering from PTSD. One of the most common approaches includes a psychotherapy approach.

The Psychotherapy Approach

Psychotherapy is a type of treatment that involves talking to a therapist in order to understand your own feelings and receive strategies to cope with your feelings and behaviors. Psychotherapy has been around for a very long time, and it can be used to treat all sorts of mental health-related issues. It's also a very popular approach to dealing with post-traumatic stress disorder. There is a wide variety of types of psychotherapy, and I want to touch on four types that are commonly used in treating PTSD. The goal of psychotherapy is to reduce your symptoms of PTSD and improve your mental and physical side effects. Many people claim that they experienced a decrease in gut-related issues after adopting a psychotherapy approach. When you're looking for a therapist who can lead you in a psychotherapeutic approach, there are a couple of things that you need to keep in mind. These are as follows:

- Ask your local doctor for a referral.

- Look for a therapist who is a member of the International Society of Traumatic Stress Studies (ISTSS).

- Interview a couple of therapists before making a final decision.

- Make sure that you choose a therapist you feel comfortable with.

Cognitive Behavioral Therapy

One of the most popular psychotherapy treatments is cognitive behavioral therapy (CBT). CBT focuses on changing the way that you think and behave toward a specific event or action. CBT is incredibly effective in treating PTSD and it can help to reduce the symptoms significantly. This type of therapy works by identifying and challenging negative thoughts and beliefs about yourself, the world, or a traumatic event. Negative thoughts can contribute to the symptoms of PTSD, and cognitive behavioral therapy aims to minimize these negative thoughts and prevent a snowball effect from taking place. CBT also focuses on teaching the patient coping skills to manage their anxiety and stress, which allows the patient to continue with everyday life. CBT is a short-term based treatment, and it lasts for roughly 12–16 weeks.

One of the techniques of CBT that helps in treating PTSD is called cognitive restructuring. During cognitive restructuring, you focus on identifying negative thoughts and beliefs and then replacing those negative thoughts with positive ones. CBT also makes use of exposure therapy which is a technique that gradually confronts the things that you're avoiding due to the traumatic event.

I once spoke to a young woman who was sexually assaulted when she went for a run near her home. Months after her attack, she couldn't bring herself to run again or even exercise at all. Her therapist helped her by encouraging her to start working out in the gym and working her way up from there.

Eventually, she started walking outside with a friend, and slowly she exposed herself to the event that traumatized her. After multiple sessions and overcoming her fears, she was finally able to run again and enjoy the sensation it gave her.

Eye Movement Desensitization and Reprocessing

Eye movement desensitization and reprocessing (EMDR) is a psychotherapy approach developed by Francine Shapiro in the early 1980s, and it focuses on breaking the loop that we get stuck in when we experience trauma. EMDR helps the patient to break the loop by stimulating different parts of the brain that allow you to move on and process the event properly. In short, EMDR involves following the therapist's finger with your eye, listening to tones, or tapping on your hands while you focus on the traumatic memory. The therapist then guides you through a series of eye movements and asks you to focus on different bodily sensations and feelings. As you do so, the memory gets processed, and you'll be able to let go of the negative emotions associated with it. EMDR has been found to be incredibly beneficial and effective in treating PTSD. EMDR therapy usually involves 8–12 sessions, and it is considered a very safe therapy. Eye movement desensitization and reprocessing can greatly reduce flashbacks, nightmares, and avoidance, as well as reduce feelings of anxiety and depression (Beason-Smith, 2022).

Acceptance and Commitment Therapy

Acceptance and commitment therapy is a type of psychotherapy that focuses on dealing with negative thoughts and feelings by accepting them (Glasofer, 2015). It makes use of mindfulness-based strategies to help people accept their thoughts and feelings instead of trying to ignore them. This type of therapy is highly beneficial and helpful in managing PTSD. The role of the therapist during acceptance and commitment therapy is to help the patient identify their values and develop a commitment to living in accordance with those values. When acceptance and commitment therapy is used to treat PTSD, the process follows six core elements:

- **Acceptance:** During the acceptance phase, the patient learns to accept their thoughts and feelings without any judgment, including the thoughts and feelings that are painful or distressing.

- **Defusion:** Defusion involves helping the patient see their thoughts as simply thoughts and not facts. It helps the patient to detach from the emotions.

- **Present moment awareness:** During this phase, the patient learns to focus on the present moment and let go of regret and worries.

- **Self-as-context:** This phase encourages the patient to see themselves separate from their thoughts and feelings. Instead of seeing themselves as being their emotions, they find who they are in their values and true identity.

- **Values:** The patient identifies their values and makes a commitment to living in accordance with those values, despite what they might be feeling or thinking.

- **Committed action:** In the final step, the patient takes steps to live in accordance with their values, even when it's hard or seems impossible.

Narrative Exposure Therapy

Narrative exposure therapy, also known as NET, is a psychotherapy approach to post-traumatic stress disorder that helps people to process their experiences and create a narrative about their lives. In other words, this therapy focuses on allowing the patient to tell their story and express their trauma in a safe space. By telling their story, they get to make sense of what happened to them and focus on moving forward. It helps immensely when dealing with PTSD to know that someone knows your story fully and completely. NET typically involves 4–12 sessions, each session lasting roughly 90 minutes. This allows the patient to express their emotions and ask for guidance from a professional. NET can be done in group sessions or one-on-one therapy, depending on the type of trauma and the preference.

These four treatment types can be highly beneficial and helpful when treating PTSD. Remember, in treating PTSD, you also take care of your physical health and specifically your gut health. However, therapy isn't the only solution to dealing with PTSD. Many people find spending time in nature the best course of therapy and treatment.

Connecting With Nature

Nature is an important need for all of us, whether we enjoy the outdoors or not. There are various benefits to connecting with nature which include both mental and physical health. Nature doesn't necessarily refer to hiking in the woods or going off the grid. Nature can also refer to your local park or even sitting in your own back garden. Nature generates various positive emotions such as being calm, experiencing joy, and a sense of peace (Mental Health Foundation, 2023). Spending time in nature creates the perfect opportunity to gain a fresh perspective on life and to process your emotions and feelings. Here are a couple of ideas for getting out in nature that will boost your mental and physical health.

Trail Hiking

Trail hiking is a great way to break away from your everyday life and explore nature a little bit more. Trail hiking allows you space to think and notice the small details about nature that you usually won't notice. It's a safe space where you can relax and where you don't have to focus on being perfect. Trail hiking can also introduce you to different parts of nature that you haven't explored before. For me, trail hiking is the perfect opportunity to gain perspective on my life and remember that I am just a small dot in a universe much bigger than me and that my problems probably won't cause the end of the world.

Man's Best Friend

If you don't enjoy spending time outside but know that it's good for you, getting a pet can be the perfect answer. Since pets require a lot of attention, you can double down on the benefits. You can take your dog for a walk or spend some time at the doggy park. This will encourage you to get out more and connect with nature in a new way. Having a pet is also a great mental health contributor since they are very sensitive to our emotions and can be a companion who doesn't ask too many questions. Having a pet friend might just be what you need to push you to go outside since you'll know that it is a responsibility.

Green Space at Home

As I said earlier, you don't need to embark into the unknown in order to spend time in nature. You can also create a little green oasis at your home if you have the facilities to do so. Whether you start a garden or plant some flowers, make sure that you have a green space available at your home where you can enjoy a sense of nature.

Spending time in nature can greatly benefit PTSD symptoms and it can also improve your gut health. Besides nature and therapy, you can also treat PTSD and gut emotions with nutritional strategies. Let's have a closer look at some nutritional strategies.

Nutritional Strategies

Since we know that nutrition contributes to our mental health, we also know that nutrition can be used to our advantage to treat symptoms of PTSD. With the right nutrition, you can reduce your stress and anxiety, which will already make a huge difference in your ability to manage your PTSD. Eating food that has high nutritional value will improve your mood significantly, and it will also boost your sleep, which can fight the sleep issues that come with PTSD. There are a couple of specific nutrients that are beneficial in treating PTSD, which include omega-3, fruits and vegetables, and lean protein.

Omega-3 Fatty Acids

Omega-3 fatty acids have been shown to reduce inflammation and improve your mood. Omega-3 is also great for treating PTSD and other mental disorders. Omega-3 can be found in fish, flaxseeds, and chia seeds. Try adding additional omega-3 to every meal you have this coming week. It doesn't have to be a lot at once, but a little bit with every meal will greatly benefit your mind and gut.

Fruits and Vegetables

Fruits and vegetables are filled with magnesium and vitamin B, both of which are highly recommended when treating PTSD and other mental health-related issues. Magnesium is a mineral that highly contributes to better sleep patterns, which is necessary when you're struggling with PTSD. Vitamin B is also a great source to manage moods and to boost your energy levels. Be sure to add loads of vegetables and fruits to your meal plan to experience the benefit of these nutrients fully.

Lean Protein

Consuming lean protein can be very helpful in managing PTSD. Lean protein can help reduce stress and anxiety, improve sleep, boost energy, and repair tissue muscles. Protein is essential in the production of serotonin and dopamine, which are also known as the happy hormones. Here are a few foods that you can eat to include lean protein in your diet:

- chicken breasts

- fish

- tofu

- eggs

- lentils

- beans

- quinoa

- Greek yogurt

Be sure to choose lean cuts of meat when you're cooking and trim down the fat that is visible. You can also add additional protein to your diet in the form of supplements and other protein-filled snacks. Speaking of supplements, that's another way that you can treat PTSD if you don't want to go another route. If therapy doesn't seem like something you're interested in and you've already spent loads of time outside, you can also focus on a holistic approach to treating PTSD by using nutritional and herbal supplements. These supplements can be used in various forms and can be quite beneficial in treating PTSD as well as other mental health issues. On top of that, most of these herbal supplements also contribute to a healthier gut, which ultimately means a healthier mind. In the next section, we'll look at five herbal and nutritional supplements that you can try to treat PTSD effectively. However, I highly recommend speaking to your local healthcare provider before using any supplements that are unknown to you or if you're also on other medications.

Herbal and Nutritional Supplements

Going for a more natural approach to treating your PTSD symptoms is totally normal and acceptable. There are a couple of ways that you can do this, which include adjusting your lifestyle and making use of some herbal and nutritional supplements.

Passionflower

The first herb that is incredibly beneficial for mental disorders is passionflower. This flowering plant has been used for centuries to treat anxiety and insomnia, and it can also improve your sleep quality. Passionflower can also aid in the treatment of PTSD by improving some of the PTSD-related symptoms. Passionflower can also be used after surgery to reduce the trauma on your body. Passionflower can be sedating, so be sure only to consume the recommended dosage. It can also cause other side effects, such as dizziness and headaches. If you start experiencing any of these symptoms, decrease the dosage or stop using it altogether until you've spoken to your healthcare provider.

Ashwagandha

Ashwagandha is another herb that can be used to treat a variety of conditions, such as anxiety, stress, and fatigue. It is also effective in helping people suffering from PTSD; however, more research is needed on the matter before it can be officially prescribed for PTSD. Ashwagandha can also increase relaxation and improve cognitive function, which can help someone with PTSD determine between what is real and what are flashbacks or hallucinations. Similarly to passionflower, this herb can cause some side effects, so if you experience dizziness or headaches, stop taking it and speak to your doctor first.

Ginkgo Biloba

Ginkgo biloba is a native tree in China that was originally used in Chinese medicine. However, there are various benefits to consuming ginkgo biloba, including improved memory and better circulation. Ginkgo biloba has been found especially beneficial in patients that suffer PTSD after car accidents. Ginkgo biloba is a natural remedy, so you might not notice the difference immediately, so be patient with the process. This herb can also improve sleep quality, reduce stress, and increase relaxation. Ginkgo biloba can be bought at most health and wellness stores.

Rhodiola Rosea

Rhodiola rosea is also known as the arctic root, and it is an adaptogenic herb that can help your body adjust to stress (The Botanical Therapist, 2018). This herb increases the performance of your neurotransmitters, which boosts the production of serotonin and dopamine. These hormones react positively in your body and regulate your mood effectively. This herb also encourages antioxidants in your body in order to fight the stress that you're experiencing. Rhodiola rosea is generally considered a safe option, but you might experience headaches and nausea.

L-Theanine

L-theanine is an amino acid found in certain tea leaves. While this amino acid isn't considered essential for human health, it has been shown to have a number of benefits. L-theanine increases the levels of GABA in your body, which is the neurotransmitter associated with feelings such as well-being and pleasure. L-theanine can also be used to increase relaxation in the body and reduce anxiety. It has been used in treating PTSD symptoms, especially when it comes to reducing stress and improving cognitive function. This supplement can be found in green tea or you can take it as a supplement form. L-theanine can also cause some drowsiness and dizziness, so be sure to speak to your doctor before consuming it with other medications.

We'll look at how hormones influence our gut a little bit more in the next chapter, so be sure to stay tuned for more helpful information on healing your gut. For now, I want to encourage you to choose one thing that you've learned in this chapter and apply it to your life immediately. Keep track of how you're feeling and how your body and mind are responding to different approaches.

Chapter 3:

The Role of Hormones:

Exploring the Gut-Mood

Connection

Hormones often get blamed for the *not-so-nice* things in life. Teenage boys with sweaty armpits? It must be hormones. Adult acne? Blame it on the hormones! Crying over a failed relationship? Don't worry, it's just hormones. While all of these examples might also be accurate (however, sometimes a teenage boy just needs a shower and some soap), hormones are also responsible for many other things in the body that are essential for our well-being. Hormones are chemical messengers produced by the glands in the endocrine system that travel through the bloodstream to get to the correct tissues and organs. While hormones often get blamed for impromptu crying sessions and throwing a tantrum, they also play a vital role in regulating a wide variety of bodily functions.

Hormones play a big role in our growth and development, which is why they're often connected to growing pains and teenage problems. However, growth hormones are responsible for stimulating growth in children. Hormones are also essential when it comes to reproduction. The reproductive system is controlled by hormones, especially sex hormones. Estrogen and progesterone are two hormones that are responsible for the menstrual cycle in women. Hormones go even beyond just the reproductive system, as they also play a vital role in your mood, as well as your immune system. Hormones regulate your mood, and they help to keep your immune system strong.

Hormones aren't the bad guys, even though we often blame them for the bad things that happen. The problem isn't actually with hormones at all—the problem comes in when hormones are out of balance. When hormones are out of balance, it can lead to a variety of health issues, including

- infertility.

- weight gain.

- mood disorders.

- sleep problems.

- osteoporosis.

Now, you might be wondering why I'm talking about hormones in a book about gut health and emotions. Well, that's because imbalanced hormones can affect your mood and your gut negatively. In this chapter, we'll look at how hormones contribute to your mood and the regulation of emotions. We'll also look at how your hormones can influence your gut health and vice versa. Of course, we'll also discuss dietary strategies to deal with hormones that are out of balance, as well as herbal remedies that are worth a try. We'll end the chapter with a couple of lifestyle strategies that contribute to healthy hormones. Are you ready to debunk the myth that hormones are the bad guys? Well, it's about time!

Understanding Hormones and Mood

There are a large variety of hormones in each and every one of us, and hormones are also different depending on your biological sex. Some of the most important hormones in the body include the following:

- **Estrogen:** Estrogen is a sex hormone that is produced in the ovaries. It plays quite a big role in regulating the menstrual cycle, enabling fertility, and producing bone health.

- **Progesterone:** This is another sex hormone produced by the ovaries, and it plays a role in regulating the menstrual cycle, pregnancy, and your mood.

- **Thyroid hormones:** This hormone is produced by the thyroid gland, and it plays a role in regulating your metabolism, heart rate, and body temperature.

- **Cortisol:** Cortisol is a stress hormone produced by the adrenal glands, and it's their job to respond to the body's stress receptors.

- **Insulin:** Insulin is a hormone produced by the pancreas that helps the body to use glucose for energy.

- **Glucagon:** This hormone is also produced by the pancreas, and it helps the body to release glucose from the liver.

Out of all of these hormones, the hormone with the largest effect on your mood is estrogen. Estrogen can highly affect your mood and it is responsible for maintaining the female reproductive hormones. During a woman's menstrual cycle, estrogen levels begin to fluctuate, and they are at their highest right before ovulation. After the ovulation period, ovulation levels start to decline, which has an impact on the mood. The first way in which estrogen affects the mood is by influencing the neurotransmitters in the brain (Golden Leaf, 2022). The neurotransmitters are chemicals in the brain that transmit signals from the nerve cells in the brain to the rest of the body. For this reason, certain hormones are connected to certain feelings. For example, dopamine is associated with feelings of happiness and well-being, while cortisol is associated with stress and anxiety. Estrogen plays a role in producing these neurotransmitters, and any change in estrogen will affect the transmitters.

Estrogen also affects your mood due to its influence on other hormones, and it influences the levels of the thyroid hormone, which plays a role in mood regulation (Golden Leaf, 2022). Estrogen is also responsible for regulating stress on the hypothalamic-pituitary-adrenal (HPI) axis. For all of these reasons, we know that estrogen plays a crucial role in mood regulation and emotional well-being. By following a healthy lifestyle and getting enough sleep, you should be able to balance your hormones fairly easily.

Another way that hormones affect our mood is by influencing the brain's reward system. The brain's reward system is involved in processing rewards and punishments, but when it's affected by the activity of hormones, the system can lead to changes in our emotional responses. For example, something that made you feel excited and accomplished today might lead you to feel unsatisfied tomorrow due to the brain's reward system. When your hormones are out of balance, it's more likely to lead to a sudden change in mood. This is often visible around the premenstrual phase, which is why many refer to PMS as the time when your mood can go from zero to one hundred real quick!

Gut Health and Hormonal Balance

Hormones also affect your gut health, and your gut can also affect the balance of your hormones. The gut and your hormones are two of the most important systems in the body, and they are closely connected, meaning they can influence one another quite severely. The gut microbiome (the trillions of bacteria in your gut) plays a large role in digestion and nutrient absorption. However, these functions can be affected by hormones that are out of balance. Since hormones are the chemical messengers that travel through the body, they can influence how well the gut does its job. For this reason, people with a gut imbalance are more likely to experience a hormonal imbalance, such as polycystic ovary syndrome and irritable bowel syndrome. There are three major ways that your gut health and hormones influence one another, which we'll look at more closely next.

The Production of Hormones

Even though many hormones are produced by glands, hormones can also be produced in the gut. Some of these hormones produced in the gut can affect the production and metabolism of other hormones. For example, serotonin is a hormone that's produced in the gut and it plays a huge role in regulating your mood, appetite, and sleep quality. When the production of serotonin is out of balance due to gut issues, it will lead to a snowball effect. Your mood will decrease, your sleep quality will worsen, and your metabolism will slow down, causing even more gut-related issues. When your gut doesn't produce these hormones, it affects the rest of the body and it slows down many of the processes. When you take active steps to improve your gut health, your hormone levels will also improve and affect the rest of your body in a positive manner.

The Absorption of Nutrients

The gut is also responsible for absorbing nutrients from food. When food enters the body and makes its way through the digestive tract, the gut extracts the nutrients that the body requires to function. These nutrients are essential for hormone production. When your body fails to absorb nutrients, it won't be able to produce the correct amount of hormones. Vitamin D is essential in the production of sex hormones, so when your gut doesn't absorb enough vitamin D from food, your sex hormones will be out of balance. Another example is the use of zinc, which is essential in the production of thyroid hormones. When these hormones are out of balance, it can lead to a variety of serious illnesses and can cause some serious damage to the gut. That is why malnourished females often stop having a menstrual cycle or experience extreme hormone imbalances.

The Effect on the Immune System

Your immune system is part of the system that regulates hormones, and the immune system can be greatly affected by the gut. In other words, when your gut health isn't as it should be, your immune system won't be able to resist inflammation and other dangers as effectively. By failing to do so, it won't regulate the balance of hormones as it should, affecting the hormonal balance. That's why certain illnesses can lead to hormonal imbalances, such as chronic inflammation. When you take good care of your gut health, you indirectly give your hormones an additional layer of security and balance due to your immune system being strong.

It's clear that your gut health, immune system, and hormonal balance are tightly connected to one another, and therefore, when you take care of one, you take care of them all. However, the opposite of that statement is also true: when you fail to take care of one of the areas, you put them all in danger. Luckily, we can take active steps to balance our hormones in various ways, including

- adjusting our diet.

- adding herbal remedies in our life.

- adjusting our lifestyle.

Many of these strategies might overlap with strategies and remedies we discussed in Chapters 1 and 2, but it's essential that we continue to look at these so that the value of them can truly sink in. I'll keep on saying it and encourage you to make changes until it happens. The more we discuss these topics, the easier it will become for you to implement these strategies practically.

Dietary Approach for Hormonal Balance

Since your gut is so closely connected to hormonal balance, it doesn't come as a surprise to learn that you can improve your hormonal balance by adjusting your diet. Your diet can play quite a significant role in balancing hormones, which we can use to our advantage. When you're aware of this fact, you'll be able to take control of your diet and use it as a tool to strengthen the balance of your hormones. Here are a couple of ways that you can use your diet to improve your hormonal balance.

Fruits and Vegetables

Fruits and vegetables that are rich in nutrients are a great way to support hormonal balance. Since hormones require specific nutrients for effective production, the best way to ensure that you have all the nutrients you need is by adding loads of vegetables and fruits to your daily diet. Some vegetables and fruits are even more nutrient dense than others, so be sure to add the following to your diet:

- berries

- citrus fruits

- apples

- bananas

- avocados

- leafy greens

- cruciferous vegetables

- broccoli

- spinach

- carrots

An easy tip to add more fruit to your diet is by placing fruit in your kitchen where you'll constantly see it. You're more likely to reach for an apple if your eye catches a bowl of them, than when you're keeping apples in the cupboard or the fridge. When you notice the fruit, your mind will be more likely to prompt you to have them as a snack or pack them in with your lunch for work. Don't rely on your cravings to lead you to healthy snacks when you're not used to consuming loads of fruit. Rather, be intentional and plan to eat specific fruits at certain times of the day.

Limit Processed Foods

The next dietary approach that you can take in order to balance your hormones is to limit processed foods as much as possible. Processed foods are often very high in sugar, artificial ingredients, and unhealthy fats which contribute to hormonal imbalance. These ingredients that are often used in processed foods can contribute to inflammation, which can disrupt the production of hormones as well as their function. Processed foods are also low in nutrients, which are essential for your well-being and hormonal balance. Inflammation is a major contributor to hormonal imbalance and by limiting the amount of processed foods that you consume, you also decrease your chances of having high inflammation levels. By limiting processed foods, you also contribute to your general gut health. Since hormones are directly connected to the gut, this contributes to healthier hormone levels. Limiting processed foods can be quite hard but you can start by reading the labels on your food when you go grocery shopping and opting to cook meals at home instead of going out to restaurants.

Limit Sugar

Limiting sugar is another way that your dietary approach can contribute to healthy hormones. Sugar has the ability to disrupt the body's natural hormone balance since it increases insulin levels, which can in turn lead to weight gain and insulin resistance. Sugar also decreases inflammation, which interferes with the production of hormones. Sugar is also highly addictive and it can cause you to crave more sugar, which then fuels the vicious cycle. Sugar also has a direct impact on certain hormones. For example, excess sugar can increase estrogen levels, which can lead to weight gain, PMS, and infertility. Sugar also disrupts testosterone levels which cause fatigue and can decrease your sex drive. Finally, sugar also impacts cortisol levels and increases cortisol production, which causes additional stress, weight gain, and sleeping issues. While removing sugar from our diet altogether isn't necessary, it's essential that we limit our sugar intake as much as possible.

Drink Plenty of Water

By drinking a lot of water, you not only take care of your overall well-being, but you specifically contribute to balancing your hormones. When your body is dehydrated, it releases vasopressin and aldosterone, which are hormones that disrupt the balance of other hormones. When you drink plenty of water, you keep these hormones in check and balance the other hormones in the meantime. Drinking water prevents the production of vasopressin and aldosterone. Water also contributes to flushing toxins from your body. Various toxins contribute to hormone imbalance, so when you stay hydrated, you enable your body to detox itself appropriately. Staying hydrated also promotes circulation, which helps the hormones travel to where they need to be. When circulation is poor, hormones can start to build up in the blood and disrupt the body's balance. Of course, drinking loads of water also contributes to healthy digestion and gut health. While the quantity of water intake differs from person to person, a good average is to aim to drink at least eight glasses of water a day.

Take Supplements

Certain supplements can aid in balancing hormones in your body. However, certain supplements can also interact with other medications, so be sure to discuss the use of supplements with your local healthcare provider if you are using other chronic medications. One of the most common supplements to aid in hormonal balance is magnesium. Magnesium is a mineral that helps regulate the production of cortisol and improves other hormone levels. Vitamin D is another common supplement that can be used to promote hormonal balance, especially in testosterone and estrogen. Other supplements that can also be used include the following:

- zinc

- vitamin B

- iodine

- ashwagandha

- Rhodiola rosea

- probiotics

- CBD oils

Using supplements isn't a substitute for medication or medical treatment, but rather an additional add-on.

Along with your dietary changes to improve your hormonal balance, you can also make use of certain herbal remedies that are beneficial in the balancing of hormones. Let's have a closer look at three specific herbal remedies that are commonly used in treating hormone imbalance.

Herbal Remedies for Hormonal Balance

Herbal remedies have been used for centuries to treat illnesses and diseases, and while some of the uses of herbs have been replaced with other modern medications, herbal remedies can still be very helpful when treating certain health concerns. One of these cases includes hormonal balance. There are three specific herbal remedies that can be incredibly beneficial to improve hormone balance: chasteberry, dong quai, and maca root.

Chasteberry

Chasteberry is a plant that can treat a variety of women's health conditions, including hormonal imbalances. Chasteberry is often used to increase the production of progesterone and decrease the production of prolactin. These two hormones often play a large role in hormone imbalances. Chasteberry is also often used to treat premenstrual syndrome symptoms and it can be effective in treating infertility. While many find using chasteberry helpful for these issues, it doesn't help everyone; in some cases, it can lead to nausea, headaches, fatigue, and irregular periods. If you make use of chasteberry and start experiencing any of these symptoms, stop consuming this herb immediately.

Dong Quai

Dong quai is another herb that has been used to treat menstrual problems and infertility for years. It balances your hormones by reducing inflammation and improving your blood flow. Dong quai can also reduce hot flashes, and it is often used to treat pain in polycystic ovary syndrome (PCOS). Dong quai can improve hormone balance by acting as an estrogen modulator which helps to balance estrogen in the body. By improving the blood flow, it actively fights against hormone build-up and decreases inflammation. Not everyone is eligible to use dong quai since it's not suited for anyone pregnant or breastfeeding, or if you have a history of blood clots or cancer. Be sure to speak to your healthcare provider before making use of this herbal remedy. Start with a small dosage and work your way up from there, but stop the consumption as soon as you experience any side effects.

Maca Root

Maca root is a plant native to Peru that is rich in vitamins, minerals, and antioxidants. Maca root can be used for various health reasons, including improved energy levels, increased libido, improved mood, and balanced hormones. Maca root has also been used to enhance fertility levels in women, and it also reduces stress. Maca root works as a hormone balancer by stimulating the hypothalamus and pituitary glands. The pituitary glands are in charge of producing hormones and regulating hormone levels throughout the body. Maca root can either increase or decrease the production of certain hormones, depending on each individual's needs. Maca root can also be used to treat menopausal symptoms such as hot flashes and night sweats. Maca root contains sterols, which are compounds that are similar to cholesterol. Sterols can aid in the production of hormones within the body and also regulate hormone levels. The antioxidants in maca root helps the body to recover after damage and remove radicals, which improves hormone production and regulation. If you want to start using maca root, try to use it consistently for six weeks before you judge the results. Maca root works best along with a healthy diet and ample exercise.

These herbal remedies might sound simple, but they can make a big difference in your daily life. Speaking of your daily life, there are also a couple of lifestyle strategies that you can implement to improve your hormone balance.

Lifestyle Strategies

While your dietary approach and herbal remedies are essential for balanced hormones, you should also adjust your lifestyle accordingly to improve your hormone balance. Certain lifestyle habits can damage your hormones, while other habits can help you to manage and maintain hormones that are balanced throughout your body, regardless of the time of the month. I specifically want to touch on three lifestyle strategies that can contribute to balanced hormones. Let's have a closer look at each of these three lifestyle strategies.

Regular Movement

The first lifestyle strategy that improves hormonal balance is movement. When you have a lifestyle that promotes regular movement, you actively enhance the hormone balance in your body by increasing endorphins. The more you move, the more endorphins will be released, which will then boost your mood. Endorphins can also aid in pain relief and they actively fight against stress. Movement also reduces insulin resistance and increases the production of sex hormones in your body. Exercise can help to increase the production of sex hormones such as testosterone and estrogen. These hormones aid in sexual function and overall health. Regular movement also contributes to reducing inflammation, which we know is a good thing when it comes to balancing hormones. The best exercises for hormonal balance include

- strength training.

- pilates.

- moderate-intensity cardio.

Manage Stress

Another lifestyle strategy that is highly beneficial for hormone balance is managing your stress appropriately. Stress can significantly impact your hormones and the more stressed we are, the more cortisol and adrenaline get produced. While these hormones are necessary in stressful situations or emergencies, they also affect the other hormones in your body. When the stress hormones overpower the other hormones in your body, it can lead to weight gain, fatigue, mood swings, and difficulty sleeping. Stress management is an important way to balance your hormones and there are many different ways that you can go about managing your stress levels. Relaxation techniques such as meditation or deep breathing exercises can help in releasing some of the stress from your body. Another method of stress management is managing your time effectively and having a healthy work-life balance. Spending time with loved ones is another popular method of managing stress in your life. When you struggle to manage your stress, you can seek help from professionals who will aid you in coming up with a plan to manage your stress accordingly. Here are a few more examples of stress management techniques:

- reading

- listening to calming music

- spending time in nature

- getting a massage

- journaling

- going for a walk

Avoid Endocrine Disruptors

The last lifestyle strategy that you can implement to ensure a healthy hormone balance is to avoid endocrine disruptors. Endocrine disruptors are chemicals that interfere with the body's natural hormone production. Endocrine disruptors can be found in many products, such as in plastics, pesticides, and personal care products. Here are a few ways that you can avoid endocrine disruptors:

- Choose organic produce as much as possible since it is grown without any pesticides.

- Avoid plastic food containers and water bottles and use glass or stainless steel instead.

- Look for products that specifically say they're BPA-free or phthalate-free.

- Avoid scented products as much as possible, since they contain a lot of endocrine disruptors.

- Filter your tap water to reduce exposure.

- Eat a healthy diet and get enough exercise.

- Drink green tea to restore the damage that endocrine disruptors might have caused.

Hormones are just another example of how the gut and the mind are connected. It's becoming clearer by the second how everything that affects our gut also affects our mind and vice versa. In the next chapter, we'll look at how we can ease our anxiety in a way that boosts our confidence. Since anxiety can cause serious gut issues, we need to also consider the impact that the mind can have on the gut. So far, we've focused on working from the gut up to the mind, but now we're switching things around and looking at how we can manage the gut by taking care of the mind. Anxiety is a very serious issue and when not managed well, it can lead to isolation due to poor social interactions. That's why it's essential that we focus on calming that inner storm in order to truly be healthy and happy from top to bottom.

Before we jump into the next chapter though, I want to encourage you to take a couple of moments and assess your own hormonal balance. While that can be tricky without a medical test, you can still take precautionary steps to ensure that your hormones remain balanced and healthy. Identify one idea or strategy from this chapter that you can start implementing today to improve your hormonal balance.

Chapter 4:

Easing Anxiety: Building Confidence in Social Interactions and Calming the Inner Storm

Anxiety seems to be a buzzword lately, thrown around lightly and used as an excuse to get out of all sorts of uncomfortable situations. However, anxiety is, in reality, very real and very serious, and more than just feeling nervous around people you don't know. I recently had a very enlightening conversation with a young woman in her mid-20s who started experiencing anxiety for the first time a couple of months prior after moving to a new city. Her husband gave up his job, and they moved across the country, excited for the change. Yet, when they arrived in the new city, she started feeling differently. She experienced bloatedness like never before, had terrible headaches, and had struggles concentrating on her work. At first, she thought she had some strange illness, but after chatting with a doctor, she realized that she was experiencing anxiety. As someone who had never struggled with anxiety before, it was as if a whole new world opened for her. "I never realized it felt this physical," she said.

That's a common misconception when it comes to anxiety. We often assume that since anxiety is considered a mental disorder, you only experience it, well, mentally. However, anxiety affects your entire body, not just your mind. In this chapter, we'll discuss anxiety and what it really entails. We'll also look at how to overcome social anxiety by discussing techniques that can help you to reduce the symptoms of anxiety. Finally, we'll also look at inner peace techniques that you can use to calm the storm raging inside of you. Understanding anxiety is essential when it comes to understanding the gut-mind connection, so let's get right into it.

Understanding Anxiety

Anxiety is a normal and healthy emotion that everyone experiences from time to time. Anxiety can serve as a warning sign that something might be wrong and requires action. However, when anxiety isn't treated, it can lead to a chronic problem that interferes with your daily life. That's then classified as an anxiety disorder. An anxiety disorder is the most common mental illness and anxiety can range from mild to severe. Anxiety can have a significant impact on a person's physical and mental health. There are different kinds of anxiety disorders, including:

- **Generalized anxiety disorder:** GAD is characterized by constant worry and finding it difficult to control your anxious thoughts. Many people with general anxiety disorder worry about a variety of things, including finances, relationships, and work.

- **Panic disorder:** Panic disorder is characterized by a sudden or intense episode of fear. These are often referred to as panic attacks and it can cause physical symptoms such as shortness of breath, chest pain, and dizziness. Panic attacks can sometimes seem like a heart attack and they're often seen as a warning sign to take better care of your mental health.

- **Social anxiety disorder:** Social anxiety disorder is the fear of social situations. People with social anxiety disorder are often worried about being embarrassed or judged by others. Social anxiety disorder often causes individuals to avoid social situations altogether or only participate in very selected situations.

- **Specific phobias:** To have a specific phobia is to have a very specific fear of a certain object or situation. Common phobias include heights, spiders, or needles. People with specific phobias may often avoid the object altogether and go out of their way to stay away from the object or situation that might cause anxiety.

- **Post-traumatic stress:** PTSD develops after a person experiences a trauma such as a natural disaster or a car accident. People with PTSD often experience flashbacks and nightmares.

Common symptoms of anxiety include feeling worried, fear, avoidance, shortness of breath, nausea, sweating, and gut-related issues. However, when you experience symptoms of anxiety, it's not a lost cause. You can get relief from anxiety through proper nutrition, mind-body techniques, as well as certain holistic remedies.

Nutrition for Anxiety Relief

What you eat can greatly influence your mood and your anxiety levels. Even though there's no one-size-fits-all diet that can cure anxiety, certain foods can greatly boost your mood while other foods should be avoided when you're experiencing signs of anxiety. Some foods contain nutrients that have been shown to have a calming effect on the mind and the body, which is why they're beneficial when it comes to anxiety relief. I want to specifically highlight three foods that will aid your anxious mind to calm down, as well as the major culprit that you should avoid when feeling anxious.

Fruits and Vegetables

We all know that fruits and vegetables are good for us, but did you know that they can lower your anxiety levels? That's because fruits and vegetables are packed with vitamins, minerals, and antioxidants. The fruits and vegetables that are specifically beneficial when it comes to anxiety are

- berries.

- leafy greens.

- citrus fruits.

- broccoli.

- brussels sprouts.

When you're anxious, you might be tempted to eat food that brings emotional comfort to you, which usually includes foods that are oily and processed. However, having a bowl of veggies will help to calm your nervous system and will benefit your anxiety levels tremendously.

Nuts and Seeds

Nuts and seeds are incredible when it comes to treating anxiety with nutrition. That's because nuts and seeds are a great source of protein, fiber, and healthy fats, all of which promote feelings of calmness. Some good sources of nuts and seeds specifically for anxiety include

- almonds.

- walnuts.

- chia seeds.

- hemp seeds.

Nuts and seeds are both great to have as a snack and to add to your meals for the day. When you feel anxious, eating some nuts and seeds can help you to calm down and the chewing motion will also help you to not clench your jaw, which is a common habit when feeling anxious.

Dark Chocolate

Dark chocolate isn't just delicious, it's also an amazing source of antioxidants and it contains magnesium. The combination of the antioxidants and the magnesium help to reduce anxiety within the body. However, sugar can increase anxiety, so be sure to choose dark chocolate that doesn't contain a lot of sugar. The best source of dark chocolate is when it has at least 70% cocoa. A lower percentage of cocoa will most likely also contain more sugar and other unhealthy fats. Not everyone is a fan of dark chocolate, and if that's the case, try having chocolate-covered nuts and seeds—getting the best of both worlds.

Limit Alcohol

Alcohol might seem like a great way to relax and take your mind off things, and it might even work in the short term. However, alcohol can worsen anxiety symptoms in the long run. The reason for this is due to the fact that alcohol is a depressant, meaning that it slows down the central nervous system. Initially, this makes you feel more relaxed, but it will increase your anxiety symptoms, leading to such things as an increased heart rate, sweating, and difficulty sleeping. Alcohol also increases your anxiety sensitivity, meaning that you are more likely to experience more anxiety in a stressful situation when you're under the influence. You are also more likely to interpret normal actions as signs of danger, affecting anxiety levels negatively. This can also lead to a vicious cycle of drinking more alcohol.

Through a balanced diet and by limiting your alcohol usage, your dietary actions can contribute to lower levels of anxiety. However, you can't rely on your diet alone. There are also many other techniques that you can try, such as mind-body techniques.

Mind-Body Techniques for Anxiety Management

Mind-body techniques can be greatly beneficial for anxiety management. Mind-body techniques are a type of complementary and alternative medicine, and they have a lot of benefits for anxiety treatment. These techniques focus on the mind-body connection, and they aim to reduce stress and promote relaxation for the mind and the body. While there are countless mind-body techniques, I want to highlight three techniques that are highly beneficial when it comes to treating and managing anxiety levels.

Guided Imagery

Guided imagery is a relaxation technique that involves using your imagination to create a calming scene. Don't worry, you don't need to be considered creative in order to make use of guided imagery. Guided imagery can be very helpful in managing anxiety since it helps you to focus on the present moment, and it distracts you from the anxious thoughts in your mind. To practice guided imagery, you need to find a quiet place where you will not be disturbed. Start by closing your eyes and taking a couple of deep breaths. Then, start to imagine a peaceful scene where you feel relaxed. Use the guided imagery to create your own little happy place where you feel calm and at peace. The beauty of guided imagery is that you can stay in your peaceful place as long as you'd like, but when you're ready to come back, you can slowly open your eyes and continue with your day. Here's an example of guided imagery:

- You're walking through the forest, and you can hear the birds chirping. The sun is playing in the leaves of the trees, casting shadows on the path. You feel the fresh air and smell the forest floor.

- As you walk, you come across a small stream, gently flowing over the rocks and pebbles. You notice how clear the water is and you decide to take off your shoes.

- You place your feet in the cold water and you feel a rush of peace calming over you. You feel the soft breeze in your hair as the cold water rushes over your feet.

- You take a deep breath, feeling calm and at peace. All your worries and stress are getting washed away by the water.

If you're interested in trying guided imagery, find a place that is calming and peaceful to you. It doesn't have to be the same image as the one I just described. Think about what makes you feel calm and peaceful and use that as inspiration.

Body Scan

A body scan is a great technique to use when you're feeling anxious. This technique is a mindfulness practice that helps you to focus on different parts of the body and notice the release of tension as you focus on a specific body part. A body scan helps you to become more aware of your body's sensations, which is incredibly helpful in reducing anxiety. In order to do a body scan, you first need to find a place where you can be alone without being disturbed by any loud noises. Find a comfortable position to sit in with your spine straight, or you can also lie down. Close your eyes and begin to focus on your breathing. Focus on slowing down your breathing, as well as breathing in nice and deep, filling your lungs completely. Notice the rise and the fall of your chest and belly as you breathe in and out. Once your breathing is settled, you can begin your body scan by either starting at your toes, or at the top of your head. Focus on one body part at a time and notice any tension or tightness that you might be experiencing in any specific body part. Breathe out and focus on relaxing those muscles. Imagine sending positive and kind energy toward a given body part and letting go of the tension. Continue the scan by focusing on every body part, from top to bottom. Notice the sensations in every body part and let go of stress you're holding in the various parts of your body. Once you reach the end, you can breathe deeply for a couple more seconds before opening your eyes. Notice how you feel and whether you're feeling less anxious and tense. Take your time to fully come out of the scan and take note of any sensations such as warmth, coolness, or pressure. A body scan can take anywhere between 5 and 10 minutes.

Breathing Exercises

Breathing exercises are a great way to manage anxiety and to regain control over your heart rate. By intentionally slowing down your breathing when you're feeling anxious, you're allowing your body to relax and your mind to take a step back and calm down the nerves. The great thing about breathing exercises is that you can do them anywhere and for as long as you want to. You don't need a lot of time or specific resources in order to make use of this calming method. There are also various breathing types that you can choose from and try out until you find one that works for you. One of my favorite breathing methods to calm down my anxious thoughts is the 4-7-8 method of breathing. To practice this breathing method, you can try the following:

- Inhale for four seconds.

- Hold your breath for seven seconds.

- Exhale for eight seconds.

You can repeat this cycle until you feel your heart slowing down. This is considered a more advanced method since it requires breath control, so if you've never done a breathing exercise before, I recommend starting with diaphragmatic breathing. Diaphragmatic breathing includes placing one hand on your belly and one on your chest. As you inhale, your belly should rise and your chest should remain fairly still, and as you exhale, your belly should fall flat and your chest should rise. Once you've mastered this type of breathing, you can try the more advanced methods.

Holistic Remedies for Anxiety

Holistic remedies for anxiety refer to natural or alternative treatments that can be used to manage your feelings of anxiety and stress. There are many holistic remedies that people believe in, some more popular than others. One of the most popular forms of holistic treatment for anxiety is drinking herbal tea. There are three specific holistic remedies that I want to introduce to you that I believe in when it comes to treating anxiety.

Lavender

Lavender is a flowering plant that many cultures use to relax. It is probably one of the most well-known scents since many products make use of lavender-scented essential oils, especially when it comes to bathroom products and candles. Lavender is often used in aromatherapy and has many benefits, including

- reducing stress and anxiety.

- improving sleep quality.

- relieving muscle tension.

- reducing headaches.

- promoting relaxation.

You can also use lavender in various ways. The most popular is to diffuse it and use the oil in your home. You can also add lavender to your bath and soak in the water for a couple of minutes. Another way is to apply lavender oil to your skin, which helps with the immediate relief of muscle tension. Finally, lavender can also be consumed in a capsule form that you can purchase from most health stores.

Lemon Balm

Another popular holistic approach is using lemon balm. Lemon balm is a herb and it works by increasing the levels of GABA in your brain. GABA is a neurotransmitter that can have a calming effect on you. Lemon balm can be taken in various ways and it has been shown to be very helpful in treating generalized anxiety disorder. Lemon balm has very few possible side effects, which is why it is such a popular holistic method of treating anxiety. You can use lemon balm to treat anxiety in the following ways:

- **Tea:** Add 1–2 teaspoons of dried lemon balm leaves and 1 cup of hot water for about 5–10 minutes. You can drink up to three cups a day.

- **Capsules:** You can find lemon balm capsules at most health stores and it's recommended that you take 300–600 mg daily.

- **Tincture:** Add 10–20 drops of lemon balm tincture to your water three times a day. If you don't like the taste, you can also add it to your juice.

- **Essential oils:** Add 2–3 drops of lemon balm essential oil to a diffuser and apply it to your temples or chest.

Passionflower

Passionflower is another popular approach to treating anxiety in a more natural way. Passionflower is a flowering plant that works similarly to lemon balm. It also increases the GABA levels in your brain, and therefore, it's a successful way of treating generalized anxiety disorder. Passionflower is a fairly safe approach, but it's important that you speak to your healthcare provider first, especially if you're on medication. You should also avoid taking passionflower if you are pregnant or if you are breastfeeding. You can use passionflower in a number of ways, including:

- **Tea:** You can make your own passionflower tea by adding 1–2 teaspoons of dried passionflower leaves in hot water and allowing it to brew for 10–15 minutes.

- **Extract:** You can also take passionflower capsule or drops. It is recommended that you stick to a daily dosage of 300–450 mg.

- **Tincture:** You can also use passionflower tincture and add 10–20 drops to your daily water. However, do not exceed 60 drops per day.

While these three holistic strategies can help to reduce your anxiety, it's essential to remember that they will not cure your anxiety. They are simply a method of managing the symptoms more effectively. When you are able to manage your symptoms, you are more likely to function better within a social situation. In the next section, we'll look at how you can boost your self-esteem in order to reduce social anxiety even more.

Boosting Your Self-Esteem

Social anxiety can be quite crippling, and it can prevent you from living your best life and interacting with your loved ones. Social anxiety is the fear of social situations, and part of that is due to being scared of being judged or evaluated negatively. A low self-esteem is often a contributing factor to social anxiety. When you have a low self-esteem, you will often have negative thoughts about yourself, and you might even believe that you're not worthy of interacting with others. Negative thoughts about yourself can quickly lead to anxiety and avoidance, causing you to isolate yourself from the world. By boosting your self-esteem, you will reduce your social anxiety. There are a number of ways that you can boost your own self-esteem, and there are three specific approaches that I want to highlight.

Expose Yourself to Fears

As contradicting as it might sound, exposing yourself to the things that you're scared of can be helpful in boosting your self-esteem. When you face your fears head-on, you will learn that you are actually capable of more than you might think. By facing your fears and overcoming them, you'll gain confidence which actively fights social anxiety. If you're afraid of public speaking, the best way to overcome it is by doing it often and practicing until you're no longer scared. However, it's essential that you start by exposing yourself to small amounts of fear at a time and gradually work your way up. For example, perhaps you shouldn't start by addressing a crowd of thousands of people, but you could still start by giving a speech to your friends and family. Here are a couple of tips for when it comes to exposing yourself to your fears:

- Start small.

- Be patient with yourself, and don't get mad when you're still feeling anxious.

- Have a support system and talk to others about your fears.

- Reward yourself when you've accomplished a first step.

Challenge Your Negative Thoughts

Negative thoughts are a major obstacle when it comes to overcoming social anxiety. They can make us feel like we're not good enough and when we believe that we're not good enough, we'll start acting accordingly and expect others to think the same way that we do. Negative thoughts can easily lead to anxiety and low self-esteem and in order to overcome this, we need to overcome and challenge our negative thoughts. Challenging your negative thoughts can be quite tricky, especially when you're not used to it. However, just like any other habit and skill, it can be learned. Challenging your negative thoughts includes the following:

- Identify the negative thoughts that you have about yourself and understand what should be considered negative thoughts.

- Once you've identified a negative thought, you should start by questioning the accuracy of the thought. Ask yourself whether what you're thinking is really true and whether it's based on fact or feeling.

- Gather evidence to refute the negative thought and to prove to yourself that the negative thought isn't true.

- Replace the negative thought with a positive one which you can then focus on whenever the negative thought pops up.

Positive Affirmations

The final method of boosting your self-esteem that we'll be discussing is the usage of positive affirmations. When it comes to positive affirmations, you are essentially training your brain to think positively about yourself. This can help with reducing negative thoughts as well, and it's another helpful step in conquering social anxiety. Positive affirmations are not as complicated as they might sound—you simply create a positive phrase that you repeat to yourself often in order to boost how you think and feel about yourself. Here are a couple of positive affirmations that you can use to improve self-esteem:

- I am worthy of love and acceptance.

- I am capable and confident.

- I am likable and approachable.

- I don't have to be scared of making a mistake.

- I am great just the way I am.

- I am safe within this social situation.

Once you've improved your self-esteem, you'll start to notice that your anxiety will be less apparent in social situations. By reducing your stress and anxiety, your gut health will also respond accordingly and improve drastically. In the next chapter, we'll look at how your gut can also influence your mood and how we can use that to our advantage by leveraging the use of vitamins. Before we get straight to it, take a moment to assess your current anxiety levels. Which of the strategies or tips in this chapter can you implement to improve your anxiety levels this week? Once you've given them some thought, be sure to also implement them accordingly. Take note of the changes you're feeling, both mentally and physically.

Chapter 5:

From Darkness to Light:

Elevating Mood Through

Vitamins

I would like to share with you the touching story of Wilma, a 55-year-old woman who had to battle depression for most of her life. As a little girl, Wilma fell in love with gymnastics, and she was determined to make a career out of it. Unfortunately, she ended up greatly hurting her back, leading to the end of her short gymnastic career at the age of 16. A couple of years later, she got married to a farmer and moved to a small town where she worked as a teacher. She lived a full and happy life, had three beautiful daughters, and became passionate about teaching. However, living on a farm can be hard work and full of uncontrollable factors. After all three daughters graduated and left the nest empty, Wilma came face-to-face with a deep sadness. She felt empty and was filled with grief over the dream she could never accomplish—being a gymnast. At the age of 50, she felt like she had no purpose. Every day was fairly similar, and even teaching didn't scratch the itch anymore. This went on for a couple of months until one morning when her alarm woke her up, she simply turned it off and rolled over. "What's the point?" she asked herself. She realized that she had no desire to get out of bed, get showered, or even eat a meal. She convinced herself that it was only temporary and that she would feel better the following day. As the next day came and went, she didn't feel any better. Wilma realized that something was deeply wrong, and with tears in her eyes, she phoned the local doctor and expressed her concern and her dark feelings.

Depression wasn't something she had ever experienced before, but as she described her symptoms to the doctor, she knew that he was right when he diagnosed her with it. Together with her doctor, they created a plan of action for her to ensure her well-being. One of the things on the action plan was increasing her vitamin intake. Like most of us, Wilma was completely unaware that vitamins and minerals contribute to our mental well-being. However, after a couple of months of prioritizing vitamins and minerals, she felt like a completely new person.

In this chapter, we'll take a closer look at how vitamins and minerals can positively contribute to our mental well-being and take us out of a place of darkness and carry us into the light. We'll look at which vitamins are beneficial and why they contribute to elevating your mood. We'll also discuss the power of magnesium and look into a couple of minerals that are highly beneficial for mental wellness. Are you ready to elevate your mood through vitamins and minerals? Let's get right to it, then!

Essential Vitamins for Emotional Wellness

Since we already discussed how your gut and mind are connected, I won't get into too much detail regarding that again. However, it's essential that we remember the importance of a balanced diet as we're working through these vitamins and minerals that are beneficial. Even when you take supplements, it's best to accompany them with a healthy, balanced diet and lifestyle. Certain vitamins play a critical role when it comes to improving your mood and supporting your mental health. There are three vitamins in particular that we should always prioritize, especially when we're going through a rough emotional time.

Vitamin B

Vitamin B is not just one thing but a group of eight vitamins that are essential when it comes to human health. Vitamin B plays a role in many bodily functions, as well as energy production, metabolism, and brain function. When you have a vitamin B deficiency, it can cause a number of mental problems, such as depression, anxiety, and fatigue. Vitamin B supplements can help to improve your emotional wellness in various ways. Since Vitamin B is involved in the production of happy hormones, such as serotonin and dopamine, the healthier your vitamin B levels are, the happier you will be. When you have a vitamin B deficiency, it can lead to anxiety as well as mood swings. Vitamin B also improves your sleep, which also contributes to lower levels of anxiety. You can either make use of vitamin B supplements, or you can add more foods that are high in vitamin B to your daily diet, such as

- fish (tuna, salmon, and halibut).

- beef.

- eggs.

- yogurt.

- nuts and seeds.

If your vitamin B levels are deficient, your doctor might encourage getting a vitamin B booster shot or adding vitamin B supplements to your daily routine. Before you start consuming a high dosage of vitamin B, be sure to talk to your doctor about it to ensure that it's safe for you to use, especially if you are also using other medications.

Vitamin C

Vitamin C is an essential nutrient that plays many essential roles in the body, one of which is emotional wellness. Vitamin C can help improve your mental health in various ways and when your vitamin C levels are low, you might experience some mood changes. Vitamin C protects you against oxidative stress, which occurs when there is an imbalance between free radicals in your body. Free radicals are molecules that can damage your cells, and by vitamin C preventing this, your neurons are safe. Another function of vitamin C is that it contributes to neurotransmitter production, which means that the levels of your happy hormones, such as serotonin and dopamine, will be higher. Most of us use vitamin C supplements when we're battling a cold, since vitamin C supports the immune system. People with higher levels of vitamin C tend to have better mental health, which is why it's a great way to boost your emotional wellness. Good sources of vitamin C include

- citrus fruits.

- strawberries.

- broccoli.

- brussels sprouts.

- sweet potatoes.

- tomatoes.

- kale.

- cantaloupe.

- papaya.

The recommended dietary allowance for vitamin C is different for adults and children. Adults require 90 mg of vitamin C daily, while children need 45 mg daily vitamin C. There are many supplements that you can use to boost your vitamin C levels, but it's essential to not go above the limit of 2,000 mg a day.

Vitamin D

The next vitamin that is greatly beneficial for your mental health is vitamin D. Vitamin D also contributes to bone health and your immune function, and vitamin D deficiency has been linked to depression and anxiety. Vitamin D plays a role in the production of serotonin, which itself plays a big role in regulating your mood. It also helps to protect your brain from damage, which prevents mental disorders. Since vitamin D is also great at reducing inflammation, your mental health will benefit greatly from higher vitamin D levels. Unfortunately, vitamin D is slightly harder to come by in natural foods than vitamin C, but you can increase your vitamin D levels by

- eating more fatty fish, egg yolks, and fortified milk.

- taking supplements to boost the levels of vitamin D in your body.

- spending time in the sun.

When you spend a lot of time in the sun, be sure to also protect your skin from burns and damage. Don't worry—sunscreen won't prevent you from receiving vitamin D from the sun.

The Power of Magnesium

Magnesium is one of the minerals that are essential for many bodily functions. In fact, some might argue that magnesium is the most important mineral since it contributes to muscle and nerve function, blood sugar control, and blood pressure regulation. Beyond all that, magnesium is also involved in the production of serotonin, which regulates your mood. When you don't have enough magnesium in your body, it can lead to anxiety and depression, and by adding magnesium supplements to your diet, you can reduce symptoms of mental disorders. Magnesium is also a great power when it comes to regulating stress hormones in the body. Once the stressful situation has passed, magnesium works to reduce cortisol levels, which reduces anxiety symptoms. Another great power of magnesium is that it can help your muscles to relax. When you're anxious or stressed, your muscles will become tense. Luckily, magnesium can reduce that stress and stiffness, which leads to treating headaches, muscle tension, and sleeping disorders. There are many ways that you can add magnesium to your diet. However, it is essential that you speak to your healthcare provider first, before making any changes to your supplement usage. Here are some other ways that you can increase your magnesium:

- You can eat foods that are rich in magnesium, such as leafy greens, vegetables, nuts, seeds, and whole grains.

- Exercise improves magnesium absorption, so if you exercise regularly, your magnesium levels should increase.

- Try to avoid or limit your caffeine and alcohol intake since both caffeine and alcohol can deplete magnesium levels.

- Managing your stress in a healthy way can also lead to improved magnesium levels since stress can deplete magnesium levels.

Mineral Support for Mental Wellness

Magnesium isn't the only mineral that can contribute to your overall mental wellness. In fact, there are a couple of other minerals that can be highly beneficial for your mental health. There are four additional minerals that I would like to introduce to you: zinc, iron, selenium, and chromium. Let's take a closer look at each of these minerals and what they bring to the table.

Zinc

Zinc is one of the minerals that you shouldn't forget about when it comes to a healthy mindset. Zinc is absolutely crucial for brain growth and development, and it also has many other body functions, such as boosting your immune system, aiding with wound healing, and protein synthesis (Montijo, 2022). Your body can't produce zinc on its own, and therefore it's up to you to provide it with all the zinc it needs. Zinc can be obtained through a variety of plant and animal foods, and you can also use it in supplement format. Zinc is also often found in various cold medications and nasal sprays. According to a study conducted in 2021, zinc elevates the levels of brain-derived neurotrophic factor in the areas of the brain that controls emotions (Montijo, 2022). When your zinc is low, these levels drop, causing anxiety and stress. Other than supplements, you can find zinc in

- red meat.

- poultry.

- chickpeas.

- eggs.

- dairy products.

Iron

Iron plays an important role in your mental health, and having too little of it can significantly impact your overall well-being. Iron is the most common nutrient deficiency, and its importance is often overlooked (Levin, 2023). While it is possible to be iron-deficient without having anemia, the deficiency itself can lead to other serious health issues. Research has connected low iron levels with depression, anxiety, and even schizophrenia (Levin, 2023). Iron is essential in producing hemoglobin, which is a protein found in red blood cells, which carries oxygen to the brain. When you lack hemoglobin, you might experience a shortness of breath, feeling fatigue, and difficulty concentrating. You can improve your iron levels by making use of supplements or adding loads of foods to your diet that are high in iron, such as

- oysters.

- beef.

- dark chicken meat.

- lentils.

- tofu.

- spinach.

- beans.

- fortified cereals.

Selenium

Selenium is a trace mineral that you can consume by eating a variety of foods. It supports healthy functioning in your body, and it also improves your metabolism and thyroid function. Selenium is needed in small amounts, but it has a large impact on your mental well-being. It is also a powerful antioxidant, which we know contributes both to the mind and the gut. Selenium fights against infections, and it contributes greatly to your immune system. Thyroid function is essential in regulating your mood, so due to the fact that selenium boosts thyroid function, it indirectly boosts your mood. People with higher levels of selenium are less likely to experience depression and anxiety than those with low levels (Kubala, 2019). You can add selenium to your diet by consuming more of the following foods:

- Brazil nuts

- tuna

- halibut

- oysters

- cod

- salmon

- wheat germ

- nut butter

- tempeh

Chromium

Chromium isn't just an element that you learned about back in school. It's also great for treating depression and diabetes. Chromium is commonly sold in capsules, powders, or multivitamins. However, there are other ways that you can add chromium to your body. Chromium is often sold as a diet supplement since it breaks down carbohydrates, fats, and proteins (Barnhart, 2022). Grape juice and broccoli are some of the foods with the highest naturally occurring chromium levels. By boosting your chromium intake, you will improve your blood sugar and regulate your emotions better. Chromium is also helpful in treating metabolic syndrome, polycystic ovary syndrome, dyslipidemia, cancer, and coronary heart disease (Barnhart, 2022). There are some side effects of chromium, including vivid dreams, mild tremors, insomnia, and weight loss. You can add chromium to your diet by increasing your intake of the following foods:

- whole grains

- mussels

- broccoli

- grapes

- beef

- egg yolks

- cranberries

- wine

- yeast extract

Nourishing the Mind With Whole Foods

As you can see, minerals and vitamins are essential for our overall health, and specifically beneficial for our mental health. While you might be tempted to go to your nearest wellness store and buy every supplement you can find, I want to encourage you to consider using foods first. While there's nothing wrong with supplements, getting these vitamins and minerals in their natural forms is more beneficial for your health and mind. There are a couple of reasons why you should aim to nourish the mind with whole foods before relying on supplements, so let's have a look at some of these reasons.

The first reason why nourishing the mind with food is better than supplements is due to the fact that whole foods contain a variety of nutrients and not just one specific mineral or vitamin. Whole foods are also more bioavailable, meaning that they can get absorbed into the body much easier and more effectively than supplements. Foods are also safer to consume than supplements since certain supplements can have side effects. Of course, there's also the benefit of taste! Food tastes better than supplements and it's more satisfying than making use of supplements. However, if your body is really struggling, you can always combine healthy whole foods with a supplement to ensure maximum efficiency.

What you eat can greatly contribute to the state of your mental health, but with these vitamins and minerals, you can boost yourself one step closer. This is just another confirmation that the gut and the mind are closely connected, and how you treat one affects how you treat the other. In the next chapter, we'll look at how we can use our gut health to contribute to bettering our sleep patterns and improving our mental well-being with enhanced sleep.

Chapter 6:

Restoring Balance: Enhancing Sleep and Emotional Well-Being Through Gut Health

Most people, myself included, spend the majority of their lives unaware that their gut influences the quality of their sleep, which in turn influences the quality of their emotional well-being. The gut-brain axis obviously connects gut health and emotional health, but that's not all it connects. Your sleep and your emotional well-being greatly influence one another. That's why it can be hard to fall asleep when you're excited or angry. The neurotransmitters that are produced in the gut to enhance your mental health are also in charge of managing the quality of your sleep. Certain hormones in the gut can also prevent you from sleeping correctly, such as cortisol—the stress hormone. I never really gave this much thought until my dear wife started experiencing severe sleeping issues. It seemed out of nowhere—she was suddenly experiencing insomnia for the first time in her life to the point where we had to seek help from other healthcare professionals.

When we realized that your gut also influences your sleep, it all made sense. Due to added work responsibilities and a health scare, my wife was under a lot of pressure and stress, which then caused the production of stress hormones in the gut, which then communicated to the mind that it was not safe to rest. It's a vicious cycle because due to a lack of sleep, your mental health will only start to deteriorate even more, which will affect your gut health, and on and on it continues. So, how do we stop the cycle? Well, that's exactly what we'll be discussing in this chapter. We can stop the cycle by addressing the three factors that are fueling the cycle:

- addressing the sleep itself

- addressing the gut

- addressing the mental well-being

So, in this chapter, we'll look at how we can address sleep by implementing strategies to optimize sleep, we'll address which foods to add or avoid to improve sleep quality, and we'll look at how to create the perfect sleep environment and routine so that your mind can be calm and relaxed.

Strategies to Optimize Your Sleep

Not getting quality sleep can be incredibly harmful to every aspect of your life. It can lead to diseases, mental health issues, and it can even be a safety concern. There are very few things as frustrating as lying in bed and trying to fall asleep when your brain or body seems to refuse to do so. I specifically want to discuss three strategies that might help you when you're in this situation to optimize your sleep.

Regular Sleep Schedule

The first step to optimizing your sleep is one that many people overlook, and that is the importance of a regular sleep schedule. Going to be at the same time every night and getting up at the same time each morning is the best way to regulate your sleep patterns. When you have a regular sleep schedule, your body will be used to it and will start to produce the correct hormones to induce sleepiness when the time comes. While it might be hard to implement this over the weekends or when you're on vacation, it's essential that you try to maintain a regular sleep schedule all throughout the week. So, resist the urge to binge-watch movies until the early morning hours over the weekend and stick to your regular sleep schedule, or at least within an hour or so of your regular sleep schedule. By sticking to a routine, you will regulate your body's natural sleep-wake cycle.

Relaxing Routine

The second step to optimizing your sleep is by creating a relaxing routine for yourself. A relaxing bedtime routine can make a big difference in the quality of sleep you're getting. If you fall asleep on the couch while still doing something else, or if you're working until right before you want to go to sleep, you haven't given your brain the opportunity to relax yet. By relaxing, you signal your mind and body that you are starting to turn off for the night and that it can start with the different processes required. A relaxing routine might look different for everyone, but here are a few general tips that can help you to relax at night:

- Only use the bedroom for sleep and intimacy. That way, when you enter the bedroom, you will feel a sense of relaxation.

- Take a shower or a bath before getting ready for bed.

- Listen to some calming music.

- Read a chapter from a book.

- Practice journaling and process your day and feelings.

- Burn a scented candle.

- Spend some downtime with your family.

Regular Exercise

This might sound contradicting, but regular exercise can significantly enhance your sleep quality. However, you should avoid exercising right before bed or close to bedtime. When you exercise too close to your bedtime, you will find it harder to fall asleep due to the endorphins. You should aim to exercise at least 30 minutes three times a week. Be sure that you don't exercise for at least three hours before going to bed. Regular exercise will burn energy which will then help you to be sleepier when it's time for bed. Exercise will also keep your heart healthy, which will improve the quality of your deep sleep periods.

Gut-Friendly Foods for Better Sleep

Not all foods are good for your gut, and in the same way, not all foods are good for your sleep. That's why it's essential that we consume foods that are beneficial for both the gut and the quality of our sleep. Luckily, there are a few options that cover both of these factors quite well. However, before we look at the gut-friendly foods that you should consume in order to improve your sleep, we first need to address the things that you should probably stay away from, to contribute to your sleep as well as your gut health.

Avoid Caffeine and Alcohol

Caffeine and alcohol are both substances that interfere with the quality of your sleep. You should avoid caffeine because it is a stimulant that can make it incredibly hard to fall asleep. Caffeine blocks the effects of adenosine, which is the neurotransmitter that makes you feel sleepy. Caffeine can stay in your system for a very long period of time, so it's best to avoid it altogether at least 10 hours before it's time to go to bed. Too much caffeine can also have an unhealthy effect on your gut and can cause bloatedness. Alcohol is another substance that you should avoid if you want to have good-quality sleep. Despite the fact that alcohol can make you feel a bit sleepy, it ultimately disrupts your sleep as the night goes on. Alcohol interferes with your REM sleep, which is the stage where mood regulation happens. It can also cause you to wake up multiple times a night. Now that we've covered the things that you should avoid, let's have a look at gut-friendly foods that will enhance your sleep.

Warm Milk

A glass of warm milk might sound like something out of a cartoon, but it can contribute to the quality of your sleep. Since milk contains the amino acid tryptophan, it encourages serotonin in the brain. Serotonin is the neurotransmitter that helps with mood regulation as well as with sleep quality. Milk also contains calcium, which helps the body to relax and fall asleep easier. Milk is also good for your gut which makes it a great option for a bedtime snack. Furthermore, milk also increases the melatonin production in your body, which is the hormone that helps to regulate your sleep-wake cycle. If you want to make your warm milk even healthier, you can try the following tips:

- Use plant-based milk if your gut is sensitive to lactose.

- Add honey to your milk to improve the flavor, but don't use too much since it can be a source of energy.

- Add some spices to your milk to promote relaxation, such as cinnamon or nutmeg.

- Add chia seeds to your milk to promote gut health.

Salmon

Salmon is a great gut-friendly food that promotes sleep since it is rich in omega-3 fatty acids, vitamin D, and tryptophan. Salmon is also a great source of protein which also contributes to your overall well-being. Protein also helps you to feel full, which prevents you from waking up in the middle of the night. You can eat salmon either cooked or raw since both ways are gut-healthy and promote quality sleep.

Bananas

Bananas are very gut-friendly and they promote sleep due to being a source of probiotics, magnesium, and tryptophan. The fructooligosaccharides in bananas (the probiotic element) promote gut health and also reduce inflammation which aids in sleep quality. The magnesium in the bananas also contributes to better sleep since it helps your body to relax.

Dark Chocolate

Dark chocolate is a delicious snack that is gut-friendly and promotes sleep. However, you need to make sure that the chocolate is 70% or more cocoa and doesn't contain a lot of sugar. You can also add dark chocolate to your warm milk to create a chocolatey drink before going to bed.

By eating these gut-friendly foods, you'll enhance your chances of good sleep significantly. However, there is more that you can do to ensure good rest other than just controlling what you eat or don't eat. One of the things that influence the quality of your sleep the most is your sleeping environment.

Creating a Sleep-Enhancing Environment

Your sleep environment can make a big difference in the quality of your sleep. Have you ever tried sleeping on a bus or an uncomfortable couch? Or maybe you've slept at a friend's house who has a dog that never stops barking! Probably not the best night's sleep you've ever had, right? That's because your sleep environment can make a huge difference in your mood, how relaxed you feel, and how deep you sleep. Here are five tips that you can implement to ensure that your sleep environment promotes quality sleep and good rest.

Comfortable Sheets and Mattresses

I used to look at beds, mattresses, and bedding and roll my eyes at how expensive they were. In fact, I thought it was useless to spend that much money on something you use only when you're asleep. How wrong I was! Investing in a quality bed and comfortable sheets is not a waste of money, especially if you consider you spend at least eight hours a day in bed! That's more time than what you typically spend in most places of your home. Make sure that you invest in sheets that you enjoy the feel of and a bed that promotes comfort and relaxation.

Dark and Cool Room

If you want to get quality sleep, you need to make sure that your room is as dark as possible. Invest in blackout curtains and make sure that all the lights that might possibly illuminate your room are turned off. If that's not possible, try sleeping with a mask on that blocks out any light that might be keeping you up. Temperature is just as important since your body will struggle to switch off when it's too hot. A cool room will help you to fall asleep faster and stay asleep throughout the night. Regulating temperature isn't always easy, but with the right sheets or a cooling system, you'll be able to get a decent night's sleep.

Noise

White, brown, and green noise are all types of ambient noise that have been shown to have benefits for sleep quality, sleep duration, focus, and general relaxation. Each type of noise has different qualities and you can choose the noise that works best for you. The type of noise will mainly depend on your preference as well as your needs.

- **White noise:** White noise is sound that contains equal amounts of energy at all frequencies. It's often described as a staticky sound, almost like a fan or a radio. White noise can be very helpful for masking unwanted sounds such as traffic noise or snoring. White noise can also help you to fall asleep faster due to the continuous frequencies. White noise is a great option if you struggle to fall asleep.

- **Brown noise:** Brown noise is a great option when you're looking to focus and concentrate on something. It makes use of a lower frequency than white noise, and it's often described as a rumbling sound, for example, the sound of a waterfall or thunder. Brown noise can be extremely beneficial in masking unwanted sounds, and for some people, it immediately puts them into a state of sleepiness.

- **Green noise:** Green noise has more energy at a midrange frequency than white noise. It can be described as a hissing sound, like the sound of crickets or even leaves rustling in the wind. Green noise is often used for relaxation sounds, and it's often heard at retreats or spas.

By making use of these tips, you'll create an environment that enhances your sleep and contributes to the quality of your sleep. Remember: Things that can hinder your sleep environment include loud noises, electronics, incorrect temperature, and light.

Holistic Remedies to Enhance Sleep

Since the gut is connected to the mind and it all works together to either enhance or disrupt your sleep quality, you can also use other holistic remedies to enhance your sleep that are helpful for both the mind and the body. Holistic remedies can work either on their own or along with the other strategies mentioned in this chapter. Naturally, for optimal results, a combination of all the strategies is advised. Many of the other holistic remedies discussed in this book will also contribute to better sleep, but there are three specific remedies that I want to suggest in order to improve the quality of your sleep.

Chamomile

Chamomile is a flowering herb that has been used for centuries since it contains many medicinal properties. Chamomile is most commonly used as a tea to enhance relaxation and sleep. That's because chamomile contains compounds that have sedative effects, such as apigenin and bisabolol. These sedatives help to calm the mind and the body, which makes it easier to fall asleep. Chamomile tea isn't the only option, as you can also add dried chamomile flowers to your pillowcase or apply chamomile essential oil to your temples and the back of your neck. Chamomile can also help you to wake up feeling refreshed and more energized since you'll get better quality deep sleep.

Valerian Root

Valerian root is a flowering plant, and it can be used to address sleeping problems. Valerian root increases the production of GABA, which calms the mind and the body by reducing anxiety and stress. When you are more relaxed, you are more likely to fall asleep easier and get decent quality sleep. Valerian root can be used to treat insomnia, and it's often prescribed as a sleep medication. When you start taking valerian root, be sure to start with a low dosage and take it at least 30 minutes before you go to bed. If you're pregnant or breastfeeding, you shouldn't consume any valerian root, and as soon as you start experiencing any side effects, stop consuming it altogether.

Essential Oils

Essential oils are a great way to promote relaxation and enhance your sleep quality. Some of the most common and beneficial essential oils are lavender, ylang-ylang, and frankincense. These oils all have a very prominent smell and are considered very floral. These scents have the ability to make you feel relaxed, and they can reduce anxiety. You can apply essential oils to your skin or add them to a diffuser. You can also add essential oils to your bath to promote maximum relaxation.

Getting quality sleep will greatly contribute to the health of your mind and your gut, which is why it shouldn't be overlooked. By using these tips, you can prepare yourself for better sleep by consuming the right foods, preparing your environment for maximum relaxation, and relaxing the mind. By doing all these things, you will take care of all the different cogs that make the wheel spin, preventing the vicious cycle from continuing. Sometimes when we struggle to sleep, we start to rely on unhealthy factors, such as social media and emotional eating. In the next chapter, we'll look at emotional eating and the role it plays in your gut-health. We'll discuss how to transform your relationship with food by promoting emotional wellness.

Chapter 7:

Conquering Emotional Eating: Transforming Your Relationship With Food for Emotional Wellness

Emotional eating is a common coping mechanism that many of us rely on when we're faced with stress and anxiety. Some people might even rely on emotional eating when they feel scared or sad. When you practice emotional eating, you aim to replace the uncomfortable emotion you're feeling with the food you're consuming. While you're eating, it might feel amazing, but the moment you stop, you feel consumed by guilt and shame, which often spirals into another emotional eating situation. Many people don't even realize that they're emotional eaters, and this is likely because emotional eating is so common and normalized. While eating an entire tub of ice cream after a breakup might help you in the moment, it probably won't mend your broken heart in the long run. Emotional eating can also greatly affect your gut health, since you'll most likely consume unhealthy foods. Never in my life have I heard of someone eating peas and broccoli when they feel emotional, am I right? If we want to truly enhance our emotional wellness, though, we need to transform our relationship with food.

In this chapter, we'll look at how we can do just that. We'll look at triggers that might cause emotional eating, as well as how to practice mindful eating instead. We'll also discuss various self-care strategies that will improve your emotional wellness so that you'll make use of other healthy coping mechanisms instead of relying on food. Before we get to it, I want you to know that if you are an emotional eater, you don't have to feel ashamed of it. The goal of this chapter is not to judge you, but to help you to live a healthier life. For a very long period in my life, I was also an emotional eater, and I didn't even realize it because the emotion I was eating wasn't something extreme—it was boredom. I always thought I was unable to sit still and not eat something. Whether it's in the car, in front of the television, or while studying, I always wanted something to eat. Only when I realized I was emotionally eating was I able to address the behavior and find a better solution for the problem. So, don't be discouraged if you are currently struggling with emotional eating—you've got this! I know that by the end of this chapter, you'll have all the tools you need to overcome emotional eating.

Identifying Triggers

The first step to overcoming emotional eating is to identify your triggers. A trigger is something that pushes you to reach for food as a source of comfort. While most emotional eating is caused by negative emotions, some emotional eating can also be triggered by positive emotions. When you feel excited after achieving a goal, you might feel tempted to celebrate with food. While there's nothing wrong with a celebratory dinner, when it's your only source of satisfaction and emotional release, it can be a big problem. Triggers can look different for every person, but there are a couple of common triggers that you should be aware of.

Stress

Stress is one of the most common emotional triggers. That is why most people eat when they're studying or watching a scary movie. When stress becomes chronic and turns into anxiety, it can cause you to rely on food as a source of comfort on a daily basis. That's because stress produces cortisol, and cortisol triggers cravings for salty, sweet, and fried foods. The reason this happens is due to the fact that these foods provide you with a burst of energy and pleasure, which replaces the stress and anxiety temporarily. The more uncontrolled stress you have in your life, the more you might rely on sugar and fast foods to get you through the day.

Stuffing Emotions

When you stuff your emotions, you are actively suppressing or denying your feelings. This can happen for a variety of reasons, including fear of judgment or feeling like you're not allowed to express negative emotions. When we fail to deal with our emotions in a healthy way and we stuff them into a box, it can trigger us to use emotional eating as an outlet. Stuffing your emotions doesn't actually get rid of them—it simply pushes them down and out of your immediate awareness. When we stuff our emotions, we place stress on our bodies which results in craving sugary and oily foods, which then leads to emotional eating. That's why it's so important that we express our emotions in a healthy way.

Boredom or Feeling Empty

Boredom or feeling empty are other ways that we can get triggered to make use of emotional eating. When we're bored, we often reach for food as our sense of entertainment, and when we feel empty, we might use food to fill the void. When we're bored, our brains start looking for stimulation. Your brain also knows that food can provide stimulation, especially when the food is sugary or fatty. Your brain associates food with pleasure, due to the dopamine that flushes the body when you enjoy food. So, when it's looking for fun, it jumps to food as the solution. In the same way, we often use food to fill an empty void in our lives. When we're feeling lonely or have a sense of longing, using food can give a sense of fulfillment for a short period of time.

Childhood Habits

Childhood habits can trigger emotional eating even when you're well into adulthood. If food was often used as a reward when you were a child, you might still see food as a positive affirmation to turn to when you're feeling down or in the mood to celebrate. In other cases, if you were restricted from eating certain foods as a young child, you might crave more of that kind of food now as an adult and you might even consume it in bulk. This can trigger an emotional eating episode where you consume more food than what is needed due to the rush it gives you.

Social Influences

Another trigger for emotional eating is social influences. When you see other people who are eating unhealthy foods or foods that look delicious, you'll probably be tempted to also eat them or at least try them. This is due to social modeling, which is the process of learning by observing others. When you see that other people are enjoying certain types of food, you'll start to connect enjoyment with that specific food. Social influences can also lead to emotional eating due to peer pressure. If you're hanging out with friends and everyone is encouraging you to have another slice of pizza even though you know you are satisfied, you might give in and eat a couple of extra slices. While not all social influences are bad, it can lead to emotional eating.

These triggers might look a little different in your life, but the basis remains the same. You might start to notice the kind of things that trigger your emotional eating, which is a great first step. The second step in overcoming emotional eating is by implementing something called mindful eating.

Mindful Eating

Mindful eating is the practice of paying attention to your food. Now, this might sound weird, but it's all about being intentional with what you're eating as well as how you're eating. What mindset do you have when you're ready to eat a meal? When you eat mindfully, you focus on a couple of things, such as emotional and physical hunger. When you practice mindful eating, you'll be able to differentiate between real hunger or whether you're simply eating due to a trigger. While practicing mindful eating, you become aware of your thoughts and feelings about certain food types which will give you a lot of insight regarding your relationship with food. Let's take a look at five ways that you can practice mindful eating.

Slow Down

The first key to mindful eating is to slow down deliberately. Due to busy schedules and hustle culture, we tend to always be on the run even when it's not necessary. That results in eating our food as quickly as possible for no reason. When we eat our food too quickly, we fail to savor the taste. With mindful eating, you should try to take time and chew every single bite. Deliberately slow down and if you feel yourself starting to rush, put down your utensils and take a couple of deep breaths before continuing. Remind yourself that you're not in a rush and that you can take your time to truly enjoy and savor the meal. When we eat quickly, we often end up getting second helpings of food due to not feeling fully satisfied.

No Distractions

The second key to mindful eating is turning away from all distractions when you're eating. I know that eating while watching television is quite common, but it often results in you eating the meal without even realizing you've finished the entire plate of food. When you're distracted, you don't focus on the taste and goodness of the meal and you might also miss your body's cues to let you know that you're reaching fullness. So, avoid being on your phone or watching television while enjoying a meal and instead, sit down at the dinner table and think about every bite.

Think About the Taste

Part of mindful eating is enjoying the taste of food. Have you ever eaten a meal so fast that you fail to recognize just how good (or bad) it tastes? It used to happen to me quite often when I would finish the food and my wife would ask me, "How was your meal?" and I would honestly have no answer. When you take time to think about the taste, you are less likely to eat too much because you'll feel satisfied with the taste. Mindful eating is about enjoying the food in front of you and not just seeing it as a means to stay alive.

Hunger and Fullness Cues

Mindful eating aims to reconnect you with your hunger and fullness cues. Your body is actually really good at communicating to you when you're full or when you're still hungry, but we often fail to listen. Ghrelin is a hormone produced in the stomach which is known as the hunger hormone. The hunger hormone will increase your appetite and signal your body that it needs food. Leptin is the hormone that is known as the fullness hormone. This hormone decreases the appetite. However, when we fail to recognize how hungry or full we are, it can lead to emotional eating or eating more than what we actually wanted to.

Emotional Hunger and Physical Hunger

The final element of mindful eating is understanding the difference between emotional hunger and physical hunger. Mindful eating will help you to understand whether what you're feeling is caused by actual hunger (ghrelin) or whether it's caused by an emotional trigger. Physical hunger is often caused by a lack of food, and you'll start to feel physical sensations such as a growling stomach, fatigue, and lightheadedness. Emotional hunger is triggered by an emotional need, and you'll feel the need to comfort yourself with food. Through mindful eating, you can slow down and ask yourself whether what you're feeling is emotional hunger or physical hunger, and if it is emotional hunger, you can decide to find a different way of managing your emotions.

Mindful eating can help you to determine other ways to manage your emotional wellness instead of relying on food. Let's have a look at a couple of self-care strategies that can also help you to manage emotions.

Self-Care Strategies for Emotional Wellness

Self-care is a great way to take care of your emotions instead of trying to eat them away. There are many ways that self-care can help, but I want to specifically highlight three strategies to manage emotional well-being.

Spend Time With Family

Spending time with family and friends is an act of self-care because they are people that you should feel safe around. Being social is a wonderful way to deal with your emotions, even when you're experiencing negative emotions. Friends and family can help you to make sense of the situation you're facing, or they can simply help remove the pressure of having to be okay. Spending time with family can also serve as a reminder to take care of yourself in order to be the best version you can be for those you love.

Journaling

Instead of hiding away from your emotions, you can decide to journal about them. When you journal what you're feeling or experiencing, you might find it easier to understand what you're going through, which can lead to a solution. Journaling your thoughts can be tricky, but it's also refreshing and rewarding, and it can provide you with a safe space to express how you're really feeling without being scared that someone might get hurt or feeling like you have to explain yourself to others. Journaling is a wonderful technique that allows you to take control of your emotions instead of trying to avoid them altogether.

Exercise

Exercise is another great way of dealing with your emotions. In fact, exercise is so beneficial that the next chapter is dedicated to the benefits of exercise on your mental well-being and your gut. When you practice movement regularly, you'll get rid of pent-up energy and emotions that might be weighing you down. Exercise also provides clarity, and it can lead to understanding yourself and others much better.

Before we move on to the next chapter and discuss the power of movement for your mind and gut, I want to encourage you to take a couple of moments and assess your own emotional well-being and your relationship with food. Are there any triggers you should be on the lookout for? Identifying triggers can be hard at first, but it's the only way you'll be able to manage your emotional eating habits effectively.

Chapter 8:

Movement for Mind and Gut:

Exercise and Physical Activity

for Emotional Wellness

I used to hate exercise. The idea of sweating like a racehorse and running miles and miles was not appealing to me at all. So, I didn't exercise at all. I was relatively healthy, so I figured that exercise wasn't that important anyway. Well, after an annual check-up from the doctor, that little bubble of mine burst quickly. I realized that if I wanted to take my health seriously, both mentally and physically, I would have to start exercising regularly. Exercise didn't only transform me physically but also mentally. Physical activity doesn't have to feel like a chore—it can actually be quite fun! Not only is it good for you, but it also provides you with endorphins that reduce your stress. Not only that, but physical activity also contributes to healthier sleep patterns, more energy, and an improved mood. Here's the best part—you don't have to run miles and miles before getting any of these benefits. In fact, even a little bit of movement and exercise can contribute to your overall well-being.

In this chapter, we'll start by looking at different types of exercises that are beneficial for emotional wellness. We'll also look at how you can practically incorporate more physical activity into your everyday schedule. We'll explore the benefits that exercise has on your gut health, and finally, we'll look at how to create our very own exercise routine that would work for us personally. Since there's no one-size-fits-all solution, you'll have the opportunity to create your own exercise routine to ensure that it works for you and is sustainable. The goal isn't to turn you into a bikini model or to train you like you're an Olympian. Instead, the goal is to have fun with the movement and enjoy the benefits that come with it. So, with that being, let's get moving and grooving!

Types of Exercise for Emotional Wellness

There are various types of exercise that can benefit your emotional wellness. While some people prefer vigorous exercise, others prefer something more moderate. No matter your level of fitness or your age, there is an exercise style that will work for you, even if it's as simple as walking in the park. On that note, we're going to look at three types of exercises that you can choose from. Don't worry, you're not limited to only one. In fact, it's highly beneficial to switch these up and try different types on different days. The three types of exercises that are the most beneficial for mental well-being are aerobic exercises, strength training, and mind-body movement.

Aerobic Exercises

Aerobic exercise is any activity that gets your heart rate up and your blood flowing. Aerobic exercise doesn't mean that you have to squeeze into tight gym pants or jump up and down, unless you want to. Aerobic exercises include activities such as running, swimming, cycling, and dancing. These types of exercises are highly beneficial for your emotional well-being, mostly because they help by reducing stress. When you make use of aerobic exercises, you release endorphins which have a mood-boosting effect. Endorphins are also natural painkillers and can help to improve your sleep. Aerobic exercises can also relieve symptoms of anxiety and depression by boosting your self-esteem and reducing feelings of isolation. When you feel negative about yourself, it affects your mental wellness significantly, which is why aerobic exercises are so great for you due to their ability to help you lose and manage a healthy weight. What I love about this type of exercise is that it doesn't feel like I'm exercising—it simply feels like I'm doing an activity that I enjoy. A couple of years ago, my wife and I started going to dancing classes, and even though it's hard work and loads of exercise, we enjoy every minute of it, and afterward, we feel energized and happy.

Strength Training

Another type of exercise that can be highly beneficial to your mental well-being is strength training. Strength training is a type of exercise that helps to build muscle and bone mass. It can also improve your balance and coordination, which contributes to overall wellness. Strength training can also improve your self-esteem by helping you feel stronger and more capable. When done regularly, strength training can reduce symptoms of anxiety and depression, helping you to manage your emotions better. Just like aerobic exercises, strength training reduces stress by releasing endorphins and boosting your mood. Strength training is a safe and effective way to improve your emotional wellness, but it's essential that you start out slowly. If you've never done strength training before, reach out to someone with experience or work with a certified personal trainer to make sure that you don't hurt yourself and do more harm than good. Strength training includes

- squats.

- push-ups.

- pull-ups.

- deadlifts.

- overhead presses.

Mind-Body Movement

The third type of exercise that is beneficial for your mental wellness is mind-body movement. Mind-body movement is a type of exercise that integrates physical activity with mental focus and awareness. It can be a powerful tool when it comes to managing emotions as well as improving your physical well-being. Mind-body movements can reduce stress, anxiety, and depression, and they can also promote feelings of happiness and calmness. There are different types of mind-body movements that you can implement in order to fully experience the benefits. One of the most common mind-body practices is Pilates, which combines physical posture and breathing exercises. Swimming is another form of mind-body movement that contributes to mental wellness. Dancing is also a form of mind-body movement. Any dancing activity can be combined with mindfulness and awareness as you intentionally become more aware of your feelings while moving your body. Mind-body movements are great at reducing stress in your mind and body as they regulate the hormones that might be causing stress. Mind-body movements also improve sleep, which actively reduces stress and promotes relaxation.

How you move isn't nearly as important as the fact that you're moving. Whatever exercise you're doing, it's surely better than nothing. So, get up and start moving and experience the boost that comes along with it. If you don't have time or the ability to spend 30 minutes a day in the gym or to focus on an exercise period each day, you can start by incorporating movement into your daily life with a little bit more effort and intentionality.

Incorporating Movement Into Your Daily Life

Have you ever considered living a very healthy and active lifestyle that doesn't involve going to the gym or picking up weights? Sounds too good to be true, right? Well, it's not! A couple of years ago, I was walking in the mall behind an elderly lady. The mall was quite busy so I knew getting past her wouldn't be easy. Immediately, I felt slightly annoyed, thinking that I would have to walk slowly. To my surprise, I had to speed up my pace to keep up with her! To prove to myself that I wasn't as unfit as I thought, I walked behind the old lady much further than where I actually wanted to go. When she finally stopped, I was out of breath and amazed by her mobility. I went up to her and we started chatting about how I had to struggle to keep up. Amazed by her speed, I asked her, "What type of exercises do you do?" She looked at me and laughed and said, "None! I just live actively." Turns out, she walks to the store every day, she gardens, and she never takes the elevator. If you want to live a more active life, here are a couple of ways that you can incorporate movement into your daily life.

Take the Stairs

The first way that you can incorporate movement into your daily life is by following that older lady's advice and taking the stairs instead of the elevator. It might seem like a nuisance at first, but taking the stairs a couple of times a day is equivalent to a short exercise. With this simple change, you can add movement and mental wellness to your life with very little extra added effort. Despite what many think, taking the stairs doesn't really take that much longer than taking the elevator. So, get up and start climbing those stairs!

Take a Walk

The next way that you can incorporate physical activity without actually going to the gym or feeling like you're working out is by taking a brisk walk. Taking a walk every day can contribute greatly to your health, both physically and mentally. Taking a walk can also be a social relaxation after a long day when you and your partner or friend do it together. A couple of years ago, my wife and I started taking walks every single evening after dinner, unless it was raining. That way, we both get to move and relax after a long day of work and really connect with one another while enjoying the endorphins. Taking a short walk can be more beneficial than spending hours in the gym and hating every second of it.

Stand Up and Move

One of the best ways to be more active in your daily life is by standing up and moving around for a bit. Instead of sending the intern to make you some coffee—get up, stretch, and make it yourself. You'll be surprised how much this movement can contribute to your physical and mental wellness. Another way to incorporate movement, if you have an office job, is by investing in a standing desk and a walking pad. That way, you can walk and work at the same time.

Dance

Dancing is another great way to get moving and live an active lifestyle. A good friend of mine has a five-minute dance party with his family every evening. No matter whether you're in a bad mood or had a terrible day, you can still get up and move around. They incorporated the dancing rule in their home to ensure that everyone gets a nice boost of endorphins, as well as connect with one another. Dancing is a fun way to get moving and get your heart rate up. You don't need to be a good dancer in order to enjoy dancing, as long as you're moving and having fun!

Park Further Away

When we go to the mall or the grocery store, we usually search for a parking space that's as close as possible. But what if you intentionally parked further away? Well, then you'll have to walk! Parking further away is an easy, low-effort way of staying active and getting in some good steps. You don't have to park on the other side of the mall, but try parking a bit further away than you usually would and get moving. Those steps might seem insignificant to you, but trust me—they add up and contribute to your overall wellness.

While movement is great for the mind, it's also wonderful for your gut health. Let's have a look at how your gut and exercise are connected.

Gut Health Benefits of Exercise

Your mind isn't the only part of your body that experiences benefits from exercise. Exercise greatly contributes to the health of your gut, which is just another reason why you should be intentional with your movement. There are four major benefits of exercise on your gut health that might serve as an additional motivation to get up and move around a bit more often. Let's have a look at these four benefits and what we can expect to happen in the gut thanks to exercise.

Increases Blood Flow

The first improvement that exercise has on the gut is increased blood flow. When you exercise and your heart rate starts to increase, it sends more blood to your muscles and to other organs, including your gut. The additional blood flow in the gut provides a more efficient way of delivering nutrients and oxygen to the cells lining the gut. These cells prevent the gut from getting damaged, and they aid in keeping you healthy. The increased blood flow helps your gut to do its job more effectively in protecting the rest of your body and sending the correct signals to the mind.

Reduces Inflammation

As we just saw, when we exercise, we provide additional blood flow to the gut. This additional blood flow also helps to reduce inflammation that might be in the blood. In other words, let's say you might have eaten something that is causing inflammation in your gut. You might feel bloated and uncomfortable due to the inflammation, but as you exercise, the inflammation is reduced and you'll feel better overall.

Reduced inflammation also prevents other illnesses from developing and it contributes to your overall well-being. Reduced inflammation can also fight against irritable bowel syndrome and inflammatory bowel disease by keeping the digestive tract healthy.

Increases Number of Beneficial Bacteria

As we discussed earlier, not all bacteria are bad. Beneficial bacteria are necessary in order to digest food properly, build an immune system, and improve your overall health. When you exercise, you increase the number of beneficial bacteria within your gut by increasing the production of fatty acids. Exercise also provides your immunity with the resources needed to destroy the unhealthy bacteria in your gut, restoring the balance between good and bad bacteria in the gut. The added blood flow also provides new blood vessels in the gut, which helps to support the growth of beneficial bacteria.

Improves Bowel Movement

The final benefit of exercise on the gut that I want to touch on is the fact that exercise improves your bowel movements. That's right: Exercise increases your gut mobility, which helps to move food through the digestive tract. When your gut mobility is stable, it prevents constipation and other possible digestive problems. Exercise also strengthens the muscles in the digestive tract which provides your colon with more strength to push stool out of the body more easily. People who exercise are less likely to suffer from constipation, and exercise is more beneficial for your gut than a fiber supplement.

As you can see, your gut can greatly benefit from some added exercise, as well as the rest of your body. So, our next step is to create an exercise routine that you'll be able to stick with. In order for an exercise plan to work, it needs to be realistic, and it must cater to your specific needs and desires. We'll then end this chapter by looking at a few ways to create an exercise routine that will actually work for you.

Creating an Exercise Routine

Creating an exercise routine doesn't have to be difficult or include hundreds of steps that'll leave you more confused than ever. A good exercise routine consists of easy-to-follow instructions, and it is specifically designed to fit your personal needs. If you don't know where to begin, you can create your own exercise routine by following these simple steps.

Pick a Time

The first thing you need to decide is the time. When do you want to exercise? Exercising is beneficial during various times of the day, but it can be tricky to find a time that'll fit into your schedule. So, pick a time that will work for you. Your time and my time might not align, and that's totally normal. Don't try to copy someone else's routine; instead, find a time that really works for you. If you know that you're more of a morning person, I suggest picking a time early in the morning since you're less likely to do it at night. However, if you're a night person, you can pick a time that's later in the day. However, remember not to exercise too close to your bedtime since that might disrupt the quality of your sleep.

Set Goals

When creating an exercise routine, you need to determine and consider your goals. If your dream goal is to run a 10-mile race, then maybe don't only create a plan that consists of strength training. Your exercise routine should fit with the goals that you have. So, before you create the routine, ask yourself what your goals are. If one of them is simply to be more healthy, then focus on a more balanced or holistic approach to exercise. If another goal is to simply enjoy movement again, make sure that you add loads of exercises filled with excitement and movements that you enjoy.

Get a Buddy

I believe everything is easier when you're not going through it alone, so reach out to a friend and ask them to join you on this new adventure of yours. Make them part of your process and plan your exercise routine together. Find something that you both enjoy and keep each other accountable to stick to the program and the times you decide on. Getting a buddy might just be the motivation that you need to keep going!

Do Something You Enjoy

Finally, when creating your routine, make sure that you choose activities that you enjoy. Movement should be fun, so if you hate running, don't add it to your routine. Be sure to really focus on the activities that you enjoy spending time on, such as tennis or swimming. Whatever it is that you enjoy, be sure to do a lot of that. It's also okay to switch things up every now and again and try different movement types when you get bored of one. As long as you enjoy what you're doing, you're improving your overall well-being and health.

Exercise is essential for our mental health as well as for our gut health, so let's not waste any more time by avoiding getting our heart rates a little higher. Movement is essential for all ages, and not just if you're in your 20s. In the next chapter, we'll look at how you can nurture your gut health and emotional well-being at all ages. We'll start by looking at how to improve gut health in infancy all the way to having a healthy lifestyle in your golden years.

Chapter 9:

Gut Health Across the Lifespan: Nurturing Emotional Well-Being From Infancy to Golden Years

There are many ways that we can contribute to our gut health, but as we grow and age, these strategies might change slightly. In this final chapter of the mind-gut connection we've been exploring together, we'll look at different strategies that can ensure gut health across all ages of your life. Taking care of your gut starts at infancy and it's essential that we take care of our gut health all the way into our golden years. So, let's not waste any time and get right to it!

Gut Health in Early Life

Gut health in early life is essential for overall health and well-being. The community of bacteria that live in the digestive tract, also known as the gut microbiota, is still in development during the early stages of life, which is why it's a critical period in shaping the microbiota and promoting long-term health. There are many factors that influence gut health during the beginning stages of life, including proper nutrition, the baby's exposure to germs, and stress on the tiny body. Since a baby can't necessarily take active steps in promoting their own gut health, it's the responsibility of the parent or the guardian to make sure that the little one's gut is healthy and set up for success.

There are a couple of strategies that can be used to promote gut health in early life. I want to focus specifically on three strategies that can make a big difference in a child's gut health and overall wellness.

- **Breastfeeding:** When you breastfeed a baby for at least six months, the baby is more likely to have strong gut health. Breast milk is the best source of nutrition for infants and it contains a variety of nutrients and prebiotics that are essential for gut health and wellness. Breast milk is much more beneficial than formula milk and it is advised to breastfeed for as long as you feel comfortable.

- **Diverse foods:** It's essential that you introduce the little one to a variety of foods early on in their life. By introducing the child to diverse foods, the infant's gut microbiota will strengthen and be able to support a variety of beneficial bacteria. Even if your little one is a picky eater, it's vital that you continue to introduce them to different types of foods that are nutrient-dense.

- **Minimizing antibiotics:** The third strategy to improve gut health in youngsters is to minimize the use of antibiotics. You should avoid using antibiotics unless necessary since antibiotics can kill off beneficial bacteria in the gut. Even though antibiotics can also get rid of other bacteria that are harmful and fight infection, they shouldn't be used when it's not absolutely necessary since they can cause long-term gut damage. When it's absolutely essential, be sure to also provide your little one with probiotics to strengthen the healthy bacteria in their gut.

Gut Health in Adolescence and Young Adulthood

We know that gut health is essential for people of all ages, but young adults and teens often neglect their gut health due to not feeling the consequences. When you're young, your immune system is stronger, so you'll feel less ill and be able to bounce back faster after experiencing the disease. However, that doesn't mean that you should take your gut for granted. During adolescence your gut microbiota is still developing, so it's vital that you take good care of your overall gut health. Your lifestyle choices can either set your gut up for success or cause damage that will last a lifetime. Let's have a look at three strategies that young adults and teens can implement to ensure a healthy gut.

- **Healthy eating habits:** Eating a healthy diet that is rich in fruits, vegetables, and fiber can promote gut health during these years of your life. Your gut microbiota requires vitamins and minerals to ensure health and a strong immunity. The best way to ensure a healthy diet is by limiting processed foods and sugary drinks, since both of those types of foods can cause a lot of damage to the bacteria in your gut. You should also aim to eat fermented foods regularly and stay properly hydrated.

- **Stress management:** Teens and young adults can also take care of their gut by managing their stress levels. Stress can be highly damaging to your gut health and it can trigger other health-related issues as well. Stress management can be done in various ways and everyone should try to find habits that contribute to stress management. Stress management also requires proper rest and getting quality sleep. As a young adult or teen, you might be tempted to skip sleep in order to do other activities that are fun, but it's essential that you take good care of your health by sleeping enough.

- **Staying active:** When you're young, you might not feel the need to exercise regularly since you still feel young and energized. However, staying active is a great way to ensure that your gut is healthy and strong. You can implement an active lifestyle during this stage of your life by participating in hobbies that are active or by joining the gym.

Gut Health in Adulthood

As we move out of the adolescent years of our lives and into proper adulthood, we might start noticing some more gut-related problems. During this stage, you start to realize that you're perhaps not as young as you used to be and that your body requires a little bit extra to keep going. Gut health is important during this age to ensure that we remain healthy as we get older. If you're not sure whether your gut is healthy or not, you'll start to notice some signs during this stage of your life. A healthy gut will result in clear skin, strong nails, healthy hair, regular bowel movements, reduced bloating, and improved mood. The same practices that were helpful toward your gut health during the early stages of adulthood are also beneficial now, but there are also other strategies that you can rely on to improve your gut.

- **Rest and relaxation:** It's absolutely vital that you rest and relax enough during adulthood. There are many stressors that might contribute to feeling anxious and you might even start to experience guilt when you're taking things slowly every now and again. However, you shouldn't feel guilty when you're resting—you should enjoy it since it contributes to your gut health. You can rest and relax by sleeping, taking time off from work, or spending time with loved ones.

- **Balanced meals:** Eating balanced meals is still incredibly important during adulthood and it's essential that you fill your diet with nutrient-dense foods. When you fail to do so, your gut will suffer the consequences and you'll start to experience various side effects of an unhealthy gut. You should focus on adding more foods to your diet that contribute to your gut health such as fruits, vegetables, and a lot of whole grains. You should also limit your intake of sugar, caffeine, alcohol, and processed foods.

- **Physical activity:** While living an active life might come easier when you're young, it can get a little bit more tricky into adulthood. It's essential that you intentionally plan on being physically active in order to really boost your gut health and contribute to your mental wellness. You can incorporate physical activity by joining a sports team or signing up for a gym class.

Gut Health in Aging

Gut health can decline with age due to a number of factors, such as changes to the gut microbiome. As we age, the composition of the gut changes, and the harmful bacteria start to increase. This can often lead to constipation, bloating, and diarrhea. As we age, the production of stomach acid can also decrease, which makes it harder to digest food properly. Certain medications that are necessary for other illnesses and diseases might also affect the gut negatively, contributing to a weakened immune system and gut problems. There are a couple of strategies that we can incorporate during the golden years to ensure that our gut remains healthy.

- **Social connections:** It might sound strange to think that social connections can contribute to your gut health, but since the mind and the gut are connected, it makes perfect sense. The gut microbiome is a complex ecosystem that is affected by our emotions and feelings. When we're connected to other people and surrounded by love and good company, our guts will respond positively. Feeling lonely and isolated can contribute to poor gut health and it can cause feelings such as depression and anxiety.

- **Mind stimulation:** Keeping your mind stimulated is another way to take care of your gut since it contributes to your overall well-being. When your mind is sharp, it will continue to send the right signals to the rest of the body, including the gut, resulting in healthier gut health and making the right decisions regarding what's good for you.

- **Movement:** Even during the golden years, movement is still essential in order to remain healthy. Your gut requires movement to produce healthy bacteria and through physical movement, you will also experience improved bowel movements. As we get older, we might not be in the mood to hit the gym every day, but we can incorporate movement in other ways, such as going for walks in the park and taking the stairs instead of the elevator.

As you can see, gut health is essential from birth to the day that we breathe our last breath. Luckily, it's not up to chance, and we get to make smart decisions to ensure that our gut remains healthy and happy, contributing to our overall well-being. As we come to the end of this chapter and our journey together, I want to encourage you to take a couple of moments to consider how you can contribute to your gut health right now in the age bracket that you find yourself in. Sometimes the small changes can make all the difference in the long term.

Conclusion:

Sustaining Emotional Well-Being: Long-Term Strategies for Mental and Gut Health

We've made it to the end of this mind-gut journey and I am so proud of the progress you've made. Even if you haven't implemented any of the practical steps yet, you've already taken an essential step toward bettering your health and that is simply by reading this book. However, now the ball is in your court—you get to decide whether this life-changing information will only remain on the pages of this book, or whether you're going to make the practical changes in your life and enhance your own mind-gut connection for the better. By taking care of your mind and your gut, you are ultimately taking care of all the areas of wellness in your life, since everything else flows from these two points in your body. If you're not sure whether you're equipped to really take care of your own mind and gut, let's recap what we've learned on this journey:

- We started by exploring the gut microbiome and how it highly influences our emotions and feelings. We discovered the connection between the gut and healing your mind and the various strategies that we can use to take care of our mind by taking care of the gut.

- In Chapter 2, we explored the power of memory and post-traumatic stress disorder and how these things affect gut health. We looked at various strategies to combat PTSD through nutrition and emotional wellness.

- Next, we looked at the power of hormones on our gut and on our mood, and how these two are closely connected to one another.

- We also discovered how to ease anxiety by building social confidence and calming the inner storm by boosting our self-esteem.

- In Chapter 5, we explored how we can manage negative emotions through nutrition and how what we consume can contribute to our mental health.

- Furthermore, we discovered how to restore the balance in our lives by enhancing our sleep quality by managing our gut health.

- Next, we looked at how to conquer emotional eating by transforming our relationship with food and embracing healthy food practices to contribute to our emotional wellness.

- In Chapter 9, we looked at the power of movement and how exercise can help us both mentally and physically.

- Finally, we looked at various strategies to take care of our gut health during all the stages of our lives, stretching from infancy to the golden years.

As you can see, you've learned so much already! You have all the information you need to really take on this journey with confidence and embrace the mind-gut connection by taking care of all the elements contributing to your well-being. However, before we say goodbye, I want to encourage you to really commit to this journey of well-being. Taking care of your health is the biggest gift you can ever give yourself, so embrace it and invest in your own mental and physical well-being. It's been an honor to journey with you and I want to thank you for giving me the opportunity to share with you what I'm passionate about. My hope is that you feel inspired and encouraged to take charge of your life and that you'll start to experience the pure goodness of the mind-gut connection.

Remember, this is a journey—so be patient with yourself if things don't change overnight. Take your time, be encouraged, and never give up. You've got this and I know that you can break free from negative emotions holding you back from living your best life!

References

Barnhart, R. (2022, January 25). *Chromium supplement: Does it help with depression?* Psych Central. https://psychcentral.com/depression/chromium-supplement#what-is-chromium

Beason-Smith, M. (2022). *Eye movement desensitization and reprocessing for PTSD.* National Center for PTSD. https://www.ptsd.va.gov/understand_tx/emdr.asp#:~:text=Eye%20Movement%20Desensitization%20and%20Reprocessing%20(EMDR)%20is%20a%20psychotherapy%E2%80%94

Glasofer, D. (2015, October 29). *Acceptance and commitment therapy (ACT) for GAD.* Verywell Mind; Verywellmind. https://www.verywellmind.com/acceptance-commitment-therapy-gad-1393175

Golden leaf. (2022, December 20). *Link between estrogen & mood: How hormones affect emotional health.* Golden Leaf Health Center. https://goldenleafhc.com/link-between-estrogen-mood-how-hormones-affect-emotional-health/#:~:text=Estrogen%20plays%20a%20crucial%20role

Kubala, J. (2019, August 20). *7 science-based health benefits of selenium.* Healthline. https://www.healthline.com/nutrition/selenium-benefits#3.-May-protect-against-heart-disease

Levin, S. (2023, May 26). *Could low iron be making your mental health symptoms worse?* Department of Psychiatry. https://medicine.umich.edu/dept/psychiatry/news/arc

hive/202305/could-low-iron-be-making-your-mental-health-symptoms-worse#:~:text=Specifically%2C%20iron%20plays%20an%20important,schizophrenia%2C%20Levin%20and%20Gattari%20write.

Mental Health Foundation. (2023). *Nature: How connecting with nature benefits our mental health.* Www.mentalhealth.org.uk. https://www.mentalhealth.org.uk/our-work/research/nature-how-connecting-nature-benefits-our-mental-health#:~:text=People%20with%20good%20nature%20connectedness%20tend%20to%20be%20happier

Montijo, S. (2022, March 28). *Zinc: How it helps anxiety and depression.* Psych Central. https://psychcentral.com/health/zinc-anxiety#defining-zinc

NCCIH. (2020, January). *Post-Traumatic stress disorder.* NCCIH. https://www.nccih.nih.gov/health/post-traumatic-stress-disorder

Ried, K., Travica, N., Dorairaj, R., & Sali, A. (2020, May). *Healing the gut naturally.* Natural Medicine Journal. https://www.naturalmedicinejournal.com/journal/healing-gut-naturally

The Botanical Therapist. (2018, March 1). *Reflexology zone: Adrenal Gland - Cortisol and stress.* The Botanical Therapist. https://thebotanicaltherapist.co.uk/blog/f/reflexology-zone-adrenal-gland---cortisol-and-stress

Valdes, A. M., Walter, J., Segal, E., & Spector, T. D. (2018). Role of the gut microbiota in nutrition and health. *BMJ, 361*(361), k2179. https://doi.org/10.1136/bmj.k2179

Printed in Great Britain
by Amazon

39179070R00079